CARE OF THE WILD FEATHERED
AND FURRED

CARE OF THE WILD
FEATHERED & FURRED
A GUIDE TO WILDLIFE HANDLING AND CARE

By
MAE HICKMAN
MAXINE GUY

Compiled and edited by
STEPHEN LEVINE

Illustrated by
DAVID HASKINS

UNITY PRESS SANTA CRUZ

1973

SECOND PRINTING   JUNE 1974

Published by UNITY PRESS
PO Box 1037, Santa Cruz, California 95061

Library of Congress Catalog Card Number: 73-76670
ISBN 0-913300-29-2 Casebound
ISBN 0-913300-26-8 Paper

Manufactured in the United States of America

Designed by CRAIG CAUGHLAN

Dedication

I would like to thank the many people who have over the last ten years during the compilation of this book given aid and encouragement: Cleveland Amory, who carried an early form of this manuscript around and attempted to find a publisher in New York some years ago; Mary Hazell Harris and Ralph and Janet Townsend of the Defenders of Wildlife; Hal and Natie Gras of the Arizona-Sonora Desert Museum. To my husband David, who was often awakened by flying squirrels bouncing on his bed, who has put up with me all these years. And particularly to the people of Tubac who have offered me the funds that have enabled me to build the aviary of which I have always dreamt. To the various wildlife services who have cared enough to send me wildlings rather than have them exterminated.

MAXINE GUY

Dedication

To my family with love and appreciation.

To my husband who footed the bills and tolerated the inconveniences of a home overrun with wildlife.

To my daughters who babysat, fed, cleaned and helped whenever they could.

To my delightful grandchildren who already show a fondness and humane feeling for all living things.

To my gentle son whose Spirit is forever free to fly the skies he loved.

MAE HICKMAN

TABLE OF CONTENTS

Introduction

Table of Contents

ILLUSTRATIONS

INTRODUCTION

This is not a definitive treatise on wildlife care; that book cannot yet be written, for not enough is yet known. These are time-tested practices and traditional techniques used in treating common wildlife problems.

The techniques described in this book will not save all the birds or animals brought to an individual involved in wildlife care. Many of the advanced tools of the technology of healing are not available to the average person. Even an experienced wildlife veterinarian is incapable of saving the majority of wildlings brought to him; 35 percent survival is considered quite high. If the reader of this book is able to save more than 20 percent of the patients he treats, he is doing very well, and with practice and patience will be of yet greater service.

A wild bird or animal that is able to be picked up, too ill or weak, or too badly injured to escape, is in great difficulty. Already shock is near, for wildlings are never picked up in the wild, seldom touched or handled except by talon or claw. There is no handling in the wild and play is on each individual's terms. To pick up a wild creature is to bring him near critical stress.

Because a wildling stays alive that does not mean he is not dying. Periodic weighing of individual patients, which is not recommended to the inexperienced, and continuous attention to droppings are the only way to tell the condition of the convalescent. Behavior may appear "normal" until death. Non-spirited, behaviorally depressed creatures usually have extremely serious problems.

It is important when a wildling has been brought in for care that one examines him carefully to estimate the extent of his injuries. Fluff the feathers, gently feel legs and wings to be sure there is no break. If a bird lives three days he has a fifty-fifty chance of survival. More than half the creatures one tends will be found dead one morning at the bottom of the cage. The care of wildlife is not to be taken lightly; it can often be a very sad experience, though there is great joy in seeing a red-tailed hawk released, wing mended, rising silently toward freedom.

Only a few birds and animals survive. Even in the wild two out of three birds die in their first year. Red-tailed hawks probably lose 90 percent of their young. Predation and genetic failures are the greatest causes of mortality in the first year. Birds are food for other animals just as other animals are food for birds. Also there are a number of parents whose genes are not quite perfect enough to allow them to provide for their young at an appropriate rate. There are parents too that don't build proper nests. Windstorms or heavy rains in spring may knock down thousands of nests. The weak succumb. Each of these creatures dies of natural causes, feeding the continuum.

Familiarize yourself with the characteristics and behavior of the species you are tending. Be certain you know which species you are dealing with. Learn proper feeding, proper release times for migrations and study general physiology to familiarize yourself with the length of time it may take an injury to heal.

Those interested in saving wildlife should pool their information. Form a local group, contact local veterinarians to ascertain if they can supply help or advice, ask if they have experience dealing with wildlife. You may find a veterinarian who is interested and willing to help, or one who would be willing to learn more. Local Humane Societies and Animal Welfare Leagues will often know those in your area involved in treating wildlife. When seeking help for an injured wildling it might be remembered that some "humane" agencies determine what is best for an animal by what is most expedient. One should not be talked into destroying an animal by those unqualified to make such decisions. Perhaps the formation of a local group, equipped to deal with wildlife problems, will offer such agencies a feasible alternative to the destruction of injured, lost and frightened wildlings.

Recent federal laws prohibit captive maintenance of essentially all native birds even for the purpose of rehabilitation and release. According to the law, permits must be obtained, and it would be wise to locate any individuals or groups nearby that offer competent, legal wildlife care.

Of course, each person will do what he thinks best, and that decision should be based on the welfare of the creature in his care. Holding wildlife in captivity is an act of moral consequence. One should give no less attention to an injured wildling than to an ailing member of one's own family. The Chinese have a proverb stating that one who saves another's life becomes responsible for that life.

Two

At a time when Americans are developing a million acres a year, destroying valuable natural habitat, anyone involved in saving wildlife will have ample opportunity to practice his discipline. Birds are constantly subjected to the "progress" of civilization, some surviving while others pass to the endangered list. There are more deer in North America now than in the time of Columbus, yet the herds are weaker and more given to disease. And with man are introduced his predator pets: the Pennsylvania State Game Commission has estimated that farm cats in that state killed eight million birds in 1972. There are some 25 million stray cats in the United States.

Human responsibility for the destruction of wildlife is not to be underestimated. Our BB guns, automobiles, insecticides and spilt fossil fuels kill millions of birds and animals. The clear cutting of hillsides and the resulting ruin of stream beds, the waste products of industry and urban sewage, all wreak havoc on natural habitats. Mankind's sprawling development, creating a heavier concentration of wild populations in smaller and smaller areas, makes botulism and contagious disease outbreaks all the more devastating.

We must also be aware of what a friend of mine calls the "Bambi syndrome" or the "how cute" attitude of many people toward wildlife. These creatures are wonderfully free and we do them no service by projecting onto them our own limitations. While domestic animals have adapted to petting and attention and seem to thrive on fireside affection, a wild creature wants most to be left alone in the wild. The abuse of taming wild creatures is evident in their often poor success in the food competition and intense predator/prey relationships which they must face upon release.

Three

This book, like any book, including the dictionary, is partly philosophy. The concern for kitchen healing has sometimes necessitated generality; for instance, the authors speak of hepatitis to indicate a variety of liver ailments which a necropsy might show indeed to be lesions or a general malfunction. Also, the authors' term "pneumonia" may indicate a wider range of respiratory distress difficulties. Indeed, a friend who has pioneered in blood chemistry, x-rays and other advanced techniques of animal husbandry, applying the methods of human medicine, has pointed out that one would need microscopic pathological evidence to make any claims of causes of death other than those by severe trauma or obvious deterioration from disease.

The book is written in the editorial "I" to allow the first person nature of the experiences to come through. None of us who put together the book is a scientist. The authors, authorities by experience, have saved thousands of birds and animals in their more than sixty years' combined experience tending wildlife. Mae Hickman and Maxine Guy met ten years ago while both were living in Virginia. They felt there was a need for a layman's guide to caring for "the multitude of wild creatures that seem, with the help quite often of the youngfry, to wind up on mother's kitchen table." For several years notes and experiences were exchanged: "It is hard to say just what belongs to whom. For the past six years the manuscript has been awaiting completion. As I finished a section it was sent on to show the work to Mae," Maxine told me.

I met Maxine Guy, and the possibilities of this book, while I was tending a wildlife sanctuary in southern Arizona three years ago. Because the authors dealt mostly with land birds, I composed, with the considerable aid of the International Bird Rescue Research Center of Berkeley, the chapters dealing with water birds. It has been an act of assimilation rather than of original creation which has allowed me to update materials contained in the original work and compile the chapters on oil spill damage, bumblefoot, Dutch duck plague, aspergillosis, and botulism. The two years that have gone into the compilation of this book have included intensive tutoring by such extraordinary experts as Mal Raff, Jim Harris, David Smith and Alice Berkner of International Bird Rescue. Also the energies of Mark Lawshe and Beth Cooper at Unity Press have greatly aided in the completion of this task. We extend our appreciation and thanks to all of those who have participated in this work, and whose work with wildlife rejoins them to the Planet Family.

STEPHEN LEVINE
Unity Press
Santa Cruz, California
1973

xv

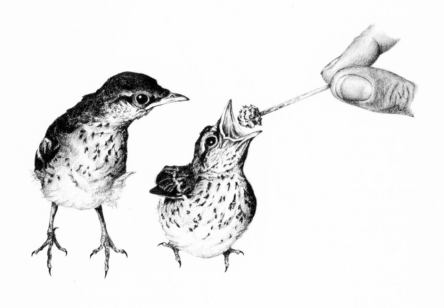

Mockingbird Fledglings

Chapter 1

CARE OF THE FEATHERED

BABY BIRDS

If you should find a baby bird on the ground, attempt to locate the nest (be sure it is the correct nest, compare the nestling you have found with the others in the nest you are considering) and then, if possible, by all means return the bird to his nest. There is no truth to the old saying that birds will reject their young if touched by human hands. They have no appreciable sense of smell.

Warmth

The first and most important step when you have a fledgling brought to you is to warm the bird as soon as possible. Nestlings, out of their nests and exposed to the elements, are highly vulnerable to death by pneumonia and need special care until they recuperate. Use a hot water bottle or heating pad (turned on low) or, if you do not have either of these, jars of hot water will do. Plastic bottles that hold liquid detergents and shampoos make excellent hot water bottles. Otherwise use glass jars. Fasten the lids tightly, wrap them in paper and snuggle the tiny birds in a nest of facial tissue directly against the jars. I suggest using two jars, one on either side of the bird, to supply more even heat to the body. The bird will benefit more from the heat if the nest is put directly on top of a padded hot water bottle or heating pad. The heating pad is really preferable to either the hot water bottle or glass jars since the latter will become cool and have to be refilled, while the heating pad will supply an even heat for as long as it is needed.

Never put a bird in the oven, leave that for your Thanksgiving turkey. It is not advisable to place one near a pilot light on top of a stove unless there is plenty of protection between the bird and the stove.

Sometimes they will be so cold that they appear lifeless, but if given the immediate benefit of warmth, they will quickly respond.

Housing

Proper homemade nests for fledglings are almost as important to their well-being as the food you give them. The parents provide a cuplike nest which serves a threefold purpose: it provides their bodies with the proper support, prevents them from falling out, and keeps them bunched together for warmth.

Tiny birds cannot stand on their legs. Their natural position is legs drawn up under their bodies and feet almost directly under their chests. In this position most of the weight of the body is centered in the back, knees, and lower stomach area. With the curved sides of the nest giving the whole body support in a semi-upright position and providing rest for the head, the bird can push against the side of the nest for balance and raise its head for food. This is the support it needs when feeding. If a proper nest is not provided the bird will sprawl, causing possible injury. Never leave a bird in this uncomfortable position.

If there are more than three fledglings to a nest, separate them into not more than three to a nest. This makes it much easier to handle them for feeding and cleaning. Birds have diaper problems, too. A bird will instinctively try to keep the nest clean by evacuating over the side. The mother bird usually removes the waste sac, so foster mother, it's your problem now. Having facial tissue handy is the easiest method of keeping the nest clean. And don't forget the problem of identifying "who was last fed?"— another good reason for splitting the group.

Small plastic berry boxes make excellent nests. I prefer them to either wooden or paper boxes. The openings in the plastic boxes allow the warmth from the incubator to circulate through the nests. These may also be easily washed if soiled.

Do not use cloth, shredded paper or cotton as nesting material. The bird's toenails are apt to get caught in cloth or cotton, and shredded paper wraps around their bodies with the chance of strangling them. However, cotton can be placed in the bottom of the box as long as tissue is placed over it in such a manner that the birds will not come in contact with the cotton. Or, use rough paper towels in the bottoms of cages. These may be placed over oiled paper. The towels give the birds traction, and the oiled paper prevents the cage bottom from becoming wet. Do not use green grass cuttings as bedding for birds or animals. It is damp and cold against their bodies.

Never wrap a baby bird in anything so that he cannot move. If you feel that he needs additional protection, lightly drop a facial tissue over him, allowing him to snuggle under for warmth or scramble out from under it if too heated or confined.

Never use old bird nests. They could and usually do have vermin in them, and soon become so soiled that they are most unsanitary. You'll have enough problems keeping them clean without adding more dirt.

Unless you are keeping the nests on an incubator which has sides, always place the nests within another box which has sides high enough to prevent the birds from falling to the floor. They will sometimes squirm over the sides of the nest (there's always one adventurer), and if they fall into another box, no harm will come to them. Cut the top and bottom out of a cardboard carton and use just the sides of the box in your incubator. There is a separate section on how to make an incubator that you will find of great value.

Never place little birds that are still in nests in the sun for warmth. Their body temperatures are high (100°-115°) and they may quickly become overheated; unable to move from the nest they will die. No bird or animal should ever be exposed to the sun while it is too small to be able to move into a shaded area.

Artificial heat for nestlings is needed only until the birds are feathered and are attempting to climb up the sides of the nest.

Feeding

Feeding should follow as soon as the bird shows signs of life and is warm and comfortable. It is most important to identify the kind of bird it is to determine the type of food to be given. Be consistent in feeding habits. It is unfair to a bird or animal to coax him to a feeder, then neglect to provide the supply of food he has come to expect.

Birds fall into two main categories: altricial and precocial. It is more than likely your patient will fall into the former group.

Birds hatched blind, naked, feeble and helpless, able only to open their beaks, defecate, and yell for food are in the altricial category. Chicks that are fully covered with down, bright-eyed and able to run after their parents and peck for their food as soon as the down dries after hatching are called precocial. Quail, ducks, chickens, grouse, and geese are in the latter category. Each category requires different care and food as well as specialized ways of feeding. If you have no bird identification book handy and the local library is too far, call the Audubon Society or a local ornithological group and describe the bird to them; they will be glad to help. Be sure your description is accurate as to size, color, markings, shape of bill, feathers (if any), legs and feet. Although it has been found that all birds eat everything, there are preferences and necessities which must be met if proper care is to be maintained.

I picked up a baby great horned owl whose care had included improper food, no log for perching, and lack of calcium. He had developed a severe case of rickets. As a result his wings were dragging. "Ricky" was put on a crash diet of bone meal, milk, prenatal care capsules, vitamins, mice, beef, and crushed chicken necks. He was skin and bones but improved with proper diet and quarters.

Never try to feed a solid diet to a baby bird that is cold and has been without food for some time. Always give warm milk with a bit of sugar added from a medicine dropper as a starter. In this way the bird can be tested to make sure it can swallow. I recommend using the glass eyedropper that has a long slender tip rather than the plastic dropper that is normally much blunter at the end. It is easier to control the quantity and avoid injuring the beak. Also, if the bird has been without food and liquid for any length of time, it may have become dehydrated, and feeding warm milk will provide both liquid and nourishment.

After you are sure that the bird can swallow, start feeding very small bites of solid food at intervals of a few minutes until it has had a good full feeding. Very young birds should be fed a soft diet. Except for pigeons, doves and hummingbirds, the foods listed below are quite sufficient. On the assumption that even a baby bird may become tired of the same food, try to supply a varied diet.

Very lean, raw ground beef is the basic food. This supplies the food values normally found in an insect diet. To the meat, add the following: hard-boiled egg yolk (one of the best foods available) mixed with baby cereal and milk or water to a consistency that may be picked up on a toothpick. For those birds who eat fruit, add scraped apple, raisins, grapes, blueberries, blackberries or raspberries that have either been mashed or cut into bite-sizes—their bite, not yours. Keep an old pair of scissors handy to cut beef, cherries, raisins or other foods to the bite sizes you want for feeding. For those birds who will later eat peanuts and sunflower seeds—like cardinals and chickadees —a small amount of peanut butter may be given twice a day.

Always give beef at each feeding, and supplement with one

or another food for variety. Also available are low-fat dog foods. At each feeding give either milk or water from a medicine dropper. Never squirt liquid down a bird's throat—always pause before giving more. Vitamins or cod liver oil should be given. Consult a veterinarian for information on the kind and amount of vitamins the bird will need each day if there is any question in your mind.

It is best to feed weak birds about every fifteen minutes for an hour or two, until they have regained their strength. Then cut the feedings to half hour intervals, then hourly. Start feeding babies about seven in the morning and continue until seven in the evening. It is not necessary to feed birds during the night. You don't see mother robin roaming around getting snacks for her young, so relax and go to bed. Parent birds start feeding at dawn and continue until dusk. They feed the babies about every fifteen minutes throughout the day, but the amount given each time will be less than the amount fed each hour by humans.

Never force a bird to eat worms. Not all birds are worm eaters. Identify the bird, get the necessary information on his natural food, then supply the nearest thing available to this. If a bird is old enough to feed himself and if identification is not possible, offer a variety of foods and learn from his selection what he prefers. Certainly if he is a worm eater the wriggle action of the worm will be sufficient to attract his attention. The three basic types of food are grain, meat, and fruit, and a variety of each should be supplied.

Normally baby birds will automatically open their beaks to be fed when you lightly tap the side of their container. The parent bird lighting on the sides of the nest is the signal that food has arrived. This movement will cause the baby to poke his head up and open his mouth wide even though his eyes may still be closed tightly. Parent birds seem to know which babies they fed last in spite of three or four gaping beaks waving and yelling to be fed. They rotate the feeding process so that each baby receives the same amount of food. To a person trying to feed a nest full of hungry birds, this array of open mouths can be very disconcerting. By the time you have fed one bird and turned to get another bite of food the birds may have changed positions and you may be uncertain about the one you fed last, so it is best to limit the birds two to a nest.

Use fingers or eyedropper for feeding once the birds are eating more solid food. A drinking straw cut on a slant is another good feeding device. It should be remembered that feeding a bird with one's fingers when it is no longer necessary to hand-feed has a tendency to make a pet of a creature, which is for that creature the end of his natural wild life. Whenever possible feed wildlings without touching them. Never use tweezers or anything made of metal. A full feeding each hour will usually be enough to sustain a young bird in good health. If the bird happens to be weak or has been injured, feed him more frequently until he has gained strength.

If a bird is a little older, with feathers and opened eyes, he may be too terrified to consider food, and may try to escape. Gently hold him and with your thumb and index finger, very gently press both sides of the base of the beak. Try it on your own mouth and you will find that your mouth will invariably open. Once the bird gets the idea that you are a source of food and mean him no harm, he will be more willing to cooperate. If a bird has been raised from a chick he will be easily feedable as he will automatically react to the sight of food or that slight tap at the side of his beak, but if he arrives too old for feeding by his parents he will not take up that relationship with you and will more likely insist on feeding himself. By all means, take care in hand-feeding. Many birds have been brought in with beaks broken from being forced open incorrectly. Care should be taken when opening a baby bird's mouth, since the beak is still soft and can easily be broken.

Even though your guest has responded to heat and food, he

still needs continued warmth and quiet. This is especially so if he lacks feathers. Steady heat helps to offset such hazards as pneumonia and the quiet helps prevent stress which would decrease his ability to survive. If the bird is feathered out and becomes too active he may be housed in a cage out of any draft with a nest of facial tissue in one corner.

Replacement of Nests Outdoors

Sometimes after heavy rains or high winds, a bird's nest will become dislodged and fall to the ground, or tipped so that the babies slide out. Usually the parent birds are frantically trying to feed and care for the babies on the ground and need help. First, if the babies have become chilled, they need to be warmed. Second, the nest will need to be replaced. Both things must be done as quickly as possible so the parent birds will not become discouraged and abandon their young. If two people are available to do the work, one should be warming the babies while the other replaces the nest. If a hot water bottle is used it can be brought out onto the lawn, covered with dry grass or leaves, and the babies placed on top of it. In this way the adult bird will see the babies and remain in the area. These methods I have found most practical in both replacing nests and reviving babies.

Often a tipped nest will need only to be leveled by securing the branch it is on to a branch above the nest. This may be done with a piece of wire or heavy cord.

To replace a nest, use a foot-square piece of hardware cloth or inch mesh chicken wire, a wire basket, or any mesh container that will allow the grass and leaves to protrude, thus giving a natural appearance. Cup the wire into a nest shape and fasten it securely in the same place as the original nest if possible. Fill the wire nest with dry, not green, leaves and grass. Be sure to wedge the grass and leaves through the wire, leaving the center of the nest cupped and leaves covering the edges of the nest. Be very sure that all the sharp edges of the wire are bent under so that young birds are not injured. Using wire allows air to come through the nest; water cannot collect in it, and it will remain reasonably dry. Portions of the old nest may be used if dry. If most of the nest is intact, simply use less leaves and grass in the wire basket and put the old nest in the center.

Do not use cardboard or wooden boxes as nest replacements. Cardboard holds water and dampness. Both of these look so unnatural that parent birds may be frightened away from them.

If the restoration of the nest and the return of the babies can be accomplished quickly and quietly with only one person or no more than two people, the parent birds will not be unduly excited and will accept and care for the babies in a man-made nest. If other people want to watch the procedure, have them remain well away from the working area and caution them to remain absolutely silent. After the babies have been replaced, go into the house and watch from a window to be sure their parents are going to cooperate. Be sure that you give the parents plenty of time to return, but don't leave the nest unattended for more than an hour. If they return, they will feed every fifteen minutes, and you will know that they have accepted your efforts. However, if they are frightened off permanently, you're a foster parent again, and good luck.

DOVES AND PIGEONS

Because of their unusual feeding habits, these birds pose a very difficult feeding problem. The young insert their beaks into the mother's mouth and she gives them a special secretion, known as pigeon's milk, from her crop (throat pouch). As the babies grow older, seeds regurgitated by the parents form a large part of their diet. One compensation is that they do not need to be fed as often as other birds, because they consume such large quantities at each feeding. I usually give four or five feedings each day, depending on the amount I feed each time.

The following procedure makes feeding simple, and the grain products and milk are nourishing and easy for the young birds to digest. Mix the following ingredients, which should be sufficient for one day's feeding, in a small bowl which can be tightly covered for refrigeration: one hard-boiled egg yolk (mashed), three tablespoons of mixed baby cereal, three tablespoons of oatmeal, three tablespoons of cornmeal. Mix with milk to a consistency quite stiff, and let it stand until the mixture becomes stiff enough to roll into bite-size pellets between the fingers. If you find that you have added too much milk, keep adding baby cereal until you reach the right consistency. Have a cup of water handy.

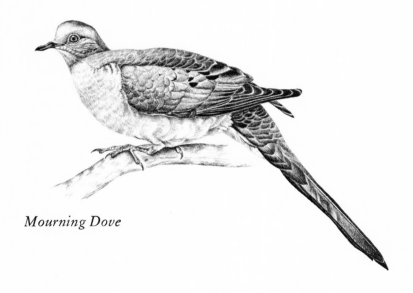

Mourning Dove

It is best to feed birds from a table that is waist high. Place the box containing the birds on the table, lay several cleaning tissues or paper towels directly in front of you, and put the bird on the tissues. Roll a small pellet of food between your fingers until it is bite size, cup your left hand over the back and wings of the bird, and with that hand gently open its mouth with thumb and forefinger. With your free hand dip the pellet quickly into the water and insert it into the bird's mouth well back in the throat. Release your hold on the bird and watch for it to swallow. This process must be repeated until the crop is well filled with food.

Baby doves have a habit of turning around in circles and flapping their wings while coaxing for food. The majority of birds usually stay in one spot and crouch down, fluttering their wings while shrieking. This circling motion by doves may be disconcerting, but if you use a waist-high table you will be able to gently draw the bird against your body to control his movements while feeding him. Dipping each pellet quickly into water before giving it to the bird will help him to swallow and will also provide some of the liquid he requires. I also give water to the bird each time I feed. Have a small container about an inch deep filled with water. Hold the container in front of the bird and gently dip his beak into the water but do not hold it there. He will soon learn to drink. Do not squirt water down a bird's throat—it may strangle him. Doves drink differently than other birds: they don't lift their heads from the water until they have had their fill, more like a cow or horse than a bird.

After the bird has had two days of feedings of the prepared mixture, try adding two tablespoons of parakeet seed to the mixture. A level teaspoon of canary gravel may be added to the mixture about once a week.

For very young birds, before they are feathered out and when they are too small to swallow the pellets of food readily, the same mixture may be given from a medicine dropper by adding a little more milk to allow it to go through the dropper easily. This will be so fluid that you can omit the water. Insert the dropper in the bird's mouth, release a few drops, remove the dropper and allow the bird to swallow. Don't rush him, watch to catch his natural rhythm then tune in and feed with him. Repeat the process until the bird has had a full feeding.

As soon as the little fellow is beginning to move around on his feet, start weaning him away from hand-feeding. Place the bird in a cage where you can observe him without distressing him, and put a small container of water in one corner. Be careful of the depth of water pans, use shallow pans in proportion to the size of the bird. Pour a generous helping of parakeet or canary seed in one corner of the cage. The bird will become curious and start pecking at the seed and before long will be quite adept. I still like to give hand-feedings for a few more days so that the accustomed supply of food is not cut off too suddenly. These gentle birds become quite spoiled and will turn around, flap their wings, and complain bitterly even after they are well able to feed themselves. Steel yourself and don't let them make a patsy out of you, although it's hard not to give in to them.

As soon as the birds are eating well, they should be transferred from the inside cage to an outside aviary where they will be protected while they learn the bird trade, picking up their own food from the ground, sunning themselves and exercising. Always remember their peculiar drinking habits and provide a drinking dish of the proper depth.

If, at the time you acquire the birds, you are not immediately able to assemble the aforementioned ingredients to feed them, give them the reliable (though temporary) standby of bread, milk and mashed egg yolk. Many other grain preparations may also be used in place of those mentioned, including wheat, wheat cereals, grits. As soon as the birds are past the stage where they need a seed as small as parakeet seed, substitute wild bird seed and/or intermediate chicken scratch.

Pigeons and collared doves have no sense of season. They will raise families in midwinter. So don't be surprised if you are

presented with a fledgling for Christmas some day. And a
Happy New Year to you, too!

NIGHTHAWKS, WHIPPOORWILLS, SWIFTS AND SWALLOWS

Use very small strips of very lean beef to feed these birds, for
moisture dipping the end of the strip in water just before feeding. This is the safest and easiest way to give liquid. The beef
strips should be very small to avoid choking. Supplement the
beef with milk from an eyedropper for the calcium that is
needed.

Here there is even more of a feeding problem than with
doves and pigeons. These little birds never pick up food from
the ground, but instead catch their meals on the wing. They are
predominantly insect eaters, so no cereal/baby food/fruit diet
for them. When they are injured and must be kept in captivity
while recuperating, they have to be hand-fed. These birds and
others of their kind fly through the air with their mouths
agape gathering insects. Lucky is the neighborhood that has a
family of swallows, swifts or any other airborne insect-
gathering bird. I even include bats in this beneficial role, in
spite of their proclivity to rabies and the fact that they are
rodents, not birds. With these swift, graceful creatures on the
wing there is no need for insect repellents.

Nighthawks sometimes become so accustomed to being hand-
fed that they run toward you with mouths open, hissing all the
while. When they have been fed their fill, they back away,
making a scolding noise while they retreat. Sometimes in their
eagerness to receive the food they grab your fingers with their
beaks, but do not flinch and startle them. They are very gentle
and easy to care for.

Baby swifts are among the most difficult to feed. They bob
their tiny heads from side to side, meanwhile setting up a con-

stant excited chatter. Since their movements are rapid, it is sometimes difficult to get the food into their mouths. The chimney swift will most probably be one kind of swift you are called upon to aid—they often get into trouble owing to their habit of building nests in chimneys. Sometimes the parent birds are killed and the little ones, when hungry, start moving around in their nests and fall down into the fireplace. Or, the nest may become dislodged and may fall with the babies within. Cover chimneys to prevent birds, squirrels and other small creatures

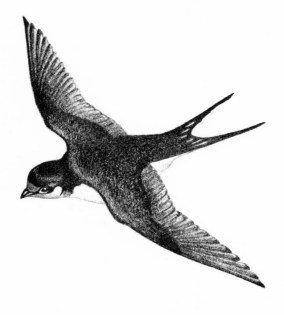

Barn Swallow

from entering. Commercially made covers may be obtained very inexpensively, or homemade covers may be cut from heavy rustproof screen.

After raising fledglings it is important to know just the right time to release them. Do not keep birds in captivity after they are able to fly well. Be sure they have ample opportunity to flex their wings and strength enough to use them before any sort of flight training. If they can fly across a room they will be able to fly much better outside. They will use air currents to their advantage as do all birds and will be able to forage for themselves. It is a good idea to release them at a time when their kinfolk are circling overhead, and they will join their family in no time. I raised three little barn swallows found in my neighborhood and the day after I released them the little "orphans" were flanked on either side on my telephone wire by the mother and father, who were most concerned about their offsprings' welfare. This is the only time, however, that I have seen parents resume care of lost children after so long an absence.

A good way to release chimney swifts is to place them on a telephone pole and stand back to watch them make their way up the pole and eventually take off. They circle in the air, gaining altitude with each circle, until they eventually seem to make up their minds what direction to take. They never come back for handouts as do some other birds, but seem to be self-sufficient once airborne.

Barn swallows are a little easier to feed and care for. The bobbing motion of the head is not so pronounced. They are quiet, docile birds and after they are old enough to perch rarely move from the log or branch provided them. In fact, one family of three babies was not kept in a cage at all, but sat on a log on the kitchen windowsill. Water was provided in a shallow container and they waddled down to the pan, bathed themselves, and then went back up on their perch. They have a very peculiar and funny waddle, these Charlie Chaplins of birdland.

HAWKS, FALCONS AND OWLS

Many times it has been my pleasure to play hostess to various predatory birds. They are most responsive to kind treatment and in no time at all can come to depend on the care and understanding of the person handling them. This trusting attitude can be a real hazard to the birds when released, since they may trust the wrong human and be killed by a hunter. Again it should be stressed that a great disservice is done any wildling by making him a pet or attributing general human emotions and responses which might eventually cost him his life.

Predatory birds are most beneficial and deserve the best treatment, but through ignorance, many are destroyed. Fortunately, some states have become aware of the imbalance of nature caused when these birds are wantonly killed and have passed laws protecting them. And now federal law protects all native birds. But much still needs to be done, both in educating the individual as to the important role played in nature by predators, and in passing laws prohibiting their capture and importation for sale in pet shops.

Meanwhile, there is a great deal to be said about the special care of these birds while guests.

Feeding predatory birds presents no problem at all. Perhaps a few forced feedings may be necessary until the bird gets accustomed to a new diet, but usually he will adapt very readily to feedings of beef, with a mouse, rat, or chicken head with the feathers left on at least twice weekly, since feathers and fur are a vital part of the diet when these birds are wild. The fur, bones and feathers act as a cleansing agent in the crop and are regurgitated as small crystalline pellets called castings. For owls, milk given from a medicine dropper is a real treat. Some of the natural food I feed to predators I am able to glean from the highways: I carry a box in my car and pick up anything that has been freshly killed. Road kills are a plentiful source of food for visiting raptors.

Beef should be lean and kept refrigerated. Beef is best but horsemeat can be substituted. Offer the food from an orange stick, chopstick, or some other small round piece of wood a few inches in length. For force feeding hawks and owls put the meat on the end of the stick and press firmly against the bird's beak, at the back just where the beak opens. When the beak opens you press the meat into the mouth and turn the stick gently. This will dislodge the meat in the bird's mouth, and if you have put it far enough into the mouth he will swallow it, but be careful not to jab the back of the throat. I have found that just a few of these forced feedings and the bird will take the meat from the stick as soon as he feels it pressed against the side of his beak. I only feed this way when the bird is sick or too frightened to pick up his food. Usually I can just hand the meat to the bird, but if frightened he may strike at your hand with his talons, so it is best not to take this chance.

I have often used a wooden paint paddle, rounded on the end. This is a good length for protection of the hands. Do not use anything metal that could cut the bird's mouth or beak. I have never had any of these birds harm me—but then I'm used to them. Cut the meat in bite-size pieces, according to the size of the bird. Feed as much as the bird wants—he'll not eat any more than he needs. For instance, a red-tailed hawk can be fed two heaping cupfuls of beef each day, once in the morning and once in the evening. A drop of vitamins plus bone meal should also be given daily.

If an adult bird is uninjured and does not require hand-feeding, place the food on a clean board on the ground and allow him to come down and make his own kill. If he is injured, place the food on the perch beside the bird. Some hawks grab the food, take it into the corner of the cage and shield it with their wings while uttering little noises of protestation as though some other bird was trying to take it away.

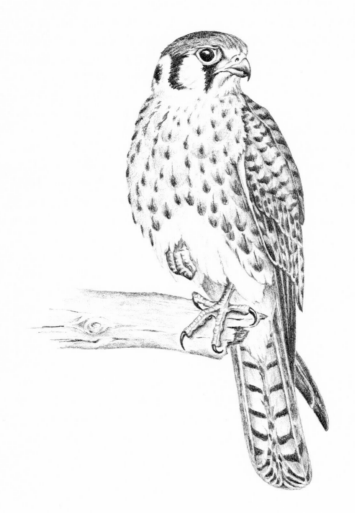

American Kestrel
(Sparrow Hawk)

Sparrow hawks prefer crickets and grasshoppers to the mice that the larger birds require. Too, dead chicks may be fed to all these predators. You might try catching a large number of grasshoppers and freezing them; just thaw them out before feeding to the birds.

Ospreys are fish eaters, but will do nicely on beef for a limited time. Fresh water provided in a pan large enough for them to bathe in is also essential.

Large hawks—red-tailed, broad-shouldered, and falcon—defecate in a different manner than do smaller birds. Instead of dropping vertically into their nest, they lean forward, lift their tail feathers, and literally *shoot* sideways out of their cage. I therefore recommend the use of cloth wrapped around that particular part of the cage they roost in, covering about half the cage between the top and bottom. All birds, if given a large enough cage, will roost in one particular part.

Predators should never be kept in small cages. They need room to move and will beat against the sides of the cage and break their feathers if it is too small. Their quarters should have one end protected on three sides and the top to prevent drafts, since they are very susceptible to pneumonia, and to restrict light, most important for night-flying owls. They need rest during the day and cannot stand bright daylight. One of the many hazards to owls is the early dawn light when the sun's rays suddenly come shooting out of the mists and strike their eyes as they wend their way home from the hunt. This blinds them temporarily and they often crash into obstacles. Telephone and electrical wires are a particular hazard to these large predators.

Hawks are often kept in pet shops in cages far too small for them to even stretch their wings. One such bird, kept on display for "atmosphere" at a miniature golf course, was forced to perch on a square rail fence, his legs tied together with rawhide thongs in such a manner that if he tried to stretch his legs, the thongs tightened. This bird was taken from the dastardly owner and cared for at length before being released. Because of the inactivity for so many weeks it was some time before he could even fly, but with care and daily exercise, he was eventually returned to the wilderness.

A perch should be provided which is large enough for a comfortable grasp by the bird's feet. Tree branches are best, and also provide a surface to sharpen the beak and razor-like talons. Don't use sandpaper on perches as it scrapes the bird's feet raw.

In captivity, and when frightened, a predator may throw back on its elbows with talons raised in self-defense. Anyone with common sense will respect these talons. They are strong and sharp enough to cut through to the bone. The bird does not fight with its beak, but with the sharp talons. Once friendly, the bird might be handled without gloves, but it is inadvisable to do so. The bird will readily step onto a gloved hand placed just behind its legs and pressed gently against the back of the legs just above the feet, allowing the bird to back onto the hand. This procedure is the opposite of the method used to coax other birds, such as robins and jays, who step forward onto a perch of any kind.

Be careful in caging birds of different species together: they may injure each other. While they may live quite harmoniously together in the wild, when caged it can be a different story. A crow, grackle, flicker, hawk or owl will probably injure or kill some of the less aggressive birds who are unable to defend themselves. Don't put a predator in a cage with any type of bird or animal that he usually preys on. Don't put two male hawks or owls in the same cage together.

When releasing predators, try to locate a large federally protected park or wildlife refuge where hunting is not allowed. Here the bird will have a chance to find food, and, although he will probably migrate from that area, hopefully he will have become wild enough by then to protect himself. Always choose good weather for releasing. There is a better chance of survival if the bird does not have a weather element to battle. Ospreys should naturally be released on a bay, river or lake where they will be able to fish for food. An open meadow with trees is ideal for releasing the sparrow hawk, who will be able to find crickets, grasshoppers and field mice there.

WATER AND WADING BIRDS

Many wading birds have been brought to me for care, and frequently they are a problem to feed. Sometimes the reason for their capture is a broken leg or wing, or injuries from gunshot. A number of them have been found soaked with waste from industrial plants. Others, for reasons which only necropsies might expose, just seem to weaken and die. One suggested cause is the presence of lead pellets from hunters mixed in with the natural food foraged in swamp and river bottoms. Another is the presence of poisons like DDT in the fish the birds eat. This was the case with a beautiful full-grown blue heron who dropped in flight a short distance from my home. He was badly toxified and died before arriving at my house with the kind people who found him.

Many of these birds, like ducks, eat grain, but those who wade and fish require a different diet. It is obvious that frogs, crustaceans and crayfish, or the seeds, greens and other native foods these birds normally eat cannot be provided easily. Since many injuries and breaks can be expected to heal within ten days to two weeks, it is reasonable to assume that a bird will not die in this length of time if it receives plenty of nourishment, even if the food is foreign to it.

For ducks and grain eaters a supply of wild bird seeds, intermediate chicken scratch (containing corn, wheat, oats and millet) plus lettuce and bread will serve nicely as a daily diet. Small quantities of moist dog food may be substituted in an emergency. Plenty of fresh water in a large, shallow pan is essential. Place the food on the ground beside the water pan: many birds will pick up the food, drop it in the water, and then eat it after it becomes soaked. Put the grain in the water pans for swans.

I have had to resort to the old standby of chunks of raw, lean beef for wading and fishing birds. Frozen fresh herring, white bait and other uncooked fish serve for gulls, terns and shore birds. I have even used canned clams for them. Most of the time the birds require hand-feeding, although in many instances as soon as the bird becomes accustomed to the new food, it can be cut into bite-size pieces and placed near the water pans for consumption. Many of these birds eat night crawlers and earthworms. Heron and American egret are most fond of this food. Drop night crawlers into the water pans and the birds will come immediately to the pan to fish for them. This is probably the nearest thing to their natural food you can provide. An electric worm catcher (there is such a thing) facilitates getting these delicacies. The earth beneath a compost pile is generally well wormed. Another trick is to soak an area and place a box or can over it; the worms will come to the surface. Usually there is someone in the vicinity who sells fishing worms, but this gets to be expensive unless you can recruit the seller to your conservation program. And don't forget the neighborhood children —they might like to help, too.

One day I received a phone call from a man who had an injured loon. The swimming pool on his property was turned into a temporary "loon pool." After a few frantic days of buying fresh fish at the pet store and dropping them into the pool, thereby depriving family and friends of a cool dip in the middle of the hot summer, he decided he needed outside help. He inquired for someone to relieve him of his responsibility. But by that time, the loon had overcome whatever had ailed him and was really living it up. After a merry chase in the pool, we were

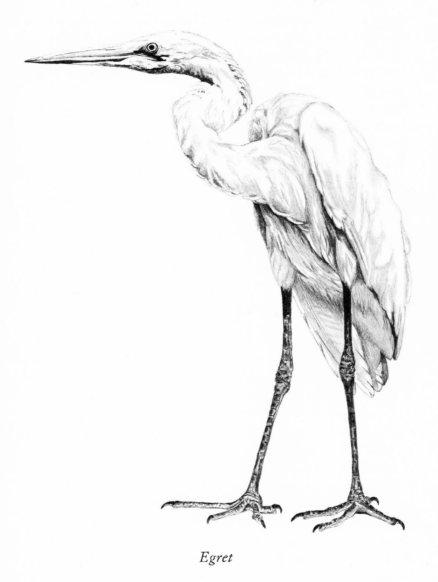

Egret

able to collect one spoiled, overfed loon and deliver him to the nearest wildlife refuge. We presume he's a lot happier there, even though the living isn't as easy.

It should be remembered that occasionally a bird trapped between walls and unreachable by hand can be helped by dropping a piece of weighted net into the enclosure so that the net reaches from the top to the area where the bird is trapped. He can use his wings to propel himself up the side if he has the net to dig his feet into.

With large birds, the hand-feeding process becomes almost a two-person job: one holds the bird while the other does the feeding. Have ready meat in elongated strips, then open the beak and place the meat well back in the bird's mouth. Hold his head gently in the air until you see him swallow. Otherwise he may shake his head and throw out the food.

Bitterns also do very nicely on raw beef. Extreme caution must be used in feeding these birds. In fright they strike out and attempt to bite. Their beaks are quite long and sharp and their necks much longer than they seem. Always reach behind the bird's neck first, gently but very firmly. Hold the bird well away from your eyes and face. Never let go of his neck while you are holding him for feeding. Feed the morsel of meat, release him until he swallows, and then repeat the process until he has completed the meal.

Always give the first feeding of meat by hand to all of these birds. Then, unless the bird is very weak and needs frequent hand-feedings, place the food near water and leave him alone to see if he will eat by himself. He will probably be frightened and won't eat if you stay near, so watch from a distance where he cannot see you. Birds may refuse to eat and allow themselves to starve. If you find that the bird does not touch the food you have left, hand-feed him at regular intervals to keep up his strength. Plenty of fresh water is necessary and a large roasting pan six inches deep serves very nicely as a water pan.

Unless a water bird is so seriously injured that it must be confined for the full length of the healing process, it is best to feed the bird and release it near the edge of a river or lake. If it is a wader, it will conceal itself in the reeds and vegetation of a swampy area and find its food there. The swimmers—ducks, gulls, grebes—will find their food by diving into a lake or river, and they are comparatively safe there. Sometimes the wings of grebes become iced during migration and they drop in fields, city streets or your backyard. One was brought in after having been found in the middle of a busy shopping area. These birds are unable to take off from a dry surface. They need water for a long, running, flapping takeoff. Grebes need a moist floor covering in their cages to prevent their feet from drying and cracking. Feed some beef and take the wayward traveler to the nearest water area and release it. Their antics in the water will amuse you and reward you for your kindness.

Since the tail is practically nonexistent on these birds, and the wings very short, many people mistakenly think that the feathers have been pulled out, thus preventing flight. It is erroneous to think that a bird cannot fly without its tail feathers, which act only as a balance and speed brake for landing. When released, grebes may immediately resume their flight, but being excellent divers, they may also dive and come up again many feet away from their point of release.

If you do not have available raw beef or grain to feed water birds, substitute bread that has been soaked in milk, or canned dog food, worms, etc. (See food substitution chart.) This cannot harm them and will provide some nourishment until you can get help for them. Again, do not keep these birds in captivity any longer than absolutely necessary. Never put them in a basement near an oil furnace—the escaping fumes may cause death even though the odor is not discernible to humans.

Whenever possible, keep the bird in a well-protected enclosure outdoors, even in winter (unless you are reading this in the northern territories of Canada). A shelter can be formed by placing a box on its side.

Ducks and geese are also fond of fresh grass and will happily graze when able to do so. Take care that the neighboring dogs are absent when walking your duck.

QUAIL, GROUSE AND OTHER PRECOCIAL BIRDS

Up to now, the birds discussed have been altricial—the help-less blind and squawking youngsters. It is equally important to know the procedures for the care of birds in the other category, the precocial birds. I have included ducks and geese in the section on water birds for the purpose of explaining diet and care, but these are really precocial, not altricial birds. The precocial birds are born with down and are able to peck and hunt for food with the parents as soon as their fluff has dried.

Quail are among the most beautiful and beneficial of these birds. I mention quail first because it is likely that you will need to care for one of them more often than other precocial birds. The tiny chicks are most appealing and seem to be irresistible to humans. After hatching, they leave the nest as soon as the down dries on their bodies. They keep close together near their parents. Their protection is the capacity to squat close to the ground and remain motionless, blending with their surroundings and becoming almost invisible. The parent bird will try to decoy danger away from the chicks, but will not abandon them, so upon discovery of a covey of chicks leave them alone. They are better able to care for themselves than any of the previously mentioned birds. Their feeding habits render a service to man; quail consume mostly insects and weed seeds.

Another characteristic of this category of birds is that their nests are built on the ground in fields, hedgerows and other low areas. Many a nest has been lost to plows, mowers or careless walkers, to say nothing of marauding cats and smallfry. Never chase or pick up young birds or animals because you think they are too young to be out of the nest. Many young wild creatures leave the nest very early. The parents usually won't approach their young while you are near, so stand well back and wait quietly and patiently for the parents to return and care for their young. If you find a young bird on the ground and see a nearby nest, be sure that the nest is the correct one before you replace the bird. If the nest belongs to another species, the parent birds may kill the intruding fledgling.

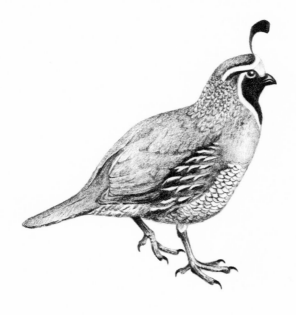

California Quail

Most people are not aware of the habits of quail chicks and upon spotting them—looking lost and forsaken, which they definitely are not—will capture them and take them home. Do not allow a child to capture and play with wild birds or animals; they are to be cherished like the children themselves. The bodies of wild creatures are not constructed to withstand constant handling, and they often die of injury or shock. Quail are very difficult to raise in captivity, so if you have one brought to you find out where it came from, take it back immediately, and let it rejoin its family. However, if you are unable to do this or know the parents have been killed, you are the foster parent.

The chicks hunt with their parents for grain and insects much as a brood of chickens will do with the mother hen. You may be able to supply the seed but you will not be able to supply the insects they need as part of their diet. A supply of wild bird seed, parakeet seed, crushed wheat and corn, hard-boiled egg yolk mixed with baby cereal, and ground beef will sustain quail chicks in captivity. They need artificial heat to take the place of the heat generated by other chicks in the family and by their parents' bodies. A heating pad under their box or incubator serves this purpose quite well. A feather duster suspended so that the tips touch the floor of the incubator gives them the feeling of security they need. They will happily snuggle under their synthetic mom.

The best policy is to leave wild chicks alone. Leave the area and let the parent birds resume their care. If quail are discovered near your home and you have a wandering cat or dog, confine your pets until the chicks have a chance to grow and move out of the area. By all means bell your cat, though cats are so stealthy in their hunting the bell may be of little help—and indeed the ringing bell does not aid nestlings or young hidden away by absent parents. Restrain cats at night, since this is the time they do the most damage.

It is also best to refrain from mentioning to small children that there is a nest nearby. Somehow, even though your own off-spring may have the kindest hearts and best intentions in the world, their friends may be unpredictable in their attitudes toward wildlife. This holds true for any kind of nest found. Children may often be unintentionally harmful because they are curious about everything and haven't, in many cases, been told how to care for the small and helpless. A living thing, so out of the ordinary, which can be carried about for friends to admire is a very attractive lure. Children often have no conception of the suffering caused by the handling and mauling of small bewildered and frightened wild creatures. So keep temptation out of sight and mind, and both beings will benefit.

HUMMINGBIRDS

These exquisite creatures are easy to feed, but over a prolonged period you will not be able to provide them a diet sufficient for their well being. In addition to the nectar from flowers they also eat millions of minute insects which the nectar attracts. I once had to keep in captivity a little female rubythroat with a crushed wing. She lived in an old dressing table which had been converted into a combination cage-incubator. This was accomplished by making one drawer the incubator, leaving the center and other drawers free from heat. In this way she could traverse the complete top of the table, using the heated area on cooler days and nights, and escaping from the heat when she wanted.

Small vials were fastened onto this cage for food and drinking water. Since she could not fly we just taped small perches and limbs to the floor of the cage. The bottom of the cage was covered either with paper towels or worn turkish towels which were stretched out over the entire bottom surface. She became quite tame and was always curious to see who entered the room. She would stretch her neck to its full length to peer over the top of the wire fence which was fastened to the outside edges of the cage.

Baby hummingbirds must be fed every fifteen to twenty minutes. If they're not fed at that interval, they won't live. I left one for about forty minutes and when I came back he was so weak he couldn't hang onto the branch. Their metabolism is so high they must be fed often and regularly. To facilitate this, make a little hummingbird carrier. Take a plastic Clorox bottle, cut out enough holes for adequate ventilation, and line the whole thing with netting. Inside, put little twigs for perching so the birds won't hurt themselves in transit. This way they can go anywhere you do, and with comfort for you both. I carried two of them to the dentist, beauty parlor, stood in receiving lines and into a box at a western rodeo where a congressman helped with the feeding. I have also seen little cages which are made in Mexico of very lightweight bamboo, and don't rattle. For small birds you can line the inside of the cage with netting to prevent them from poking their heads through the bars. The cages are also very easy to clean—just scrub them out. Never transport a bird or small animal in a cardboard carton or cage without first putting something on the bottom of the box for the creature to cling to.

Hummingbirds literally hibernate at night. Their body temperature drops considerably—you can touch them and they'll let out a tiny squeak, but they won't move. When their body temperature rises again in the morning you once again start feeding.

Sugar, honey or molasses can be added to water to serve as temporary food for the hummingbird, but this is not enough variety for prolonged feeding. Some researchers have found that honey is not an ideal substance for feeders since it acts as a medium for the growth of a harmful fungus, so sugar is preferred. Sometimes the bird's mouth will need to be opened gently and liquid dropped in to start the feeding process, but this must be done very carefully so that the bird does not strangle. Give a drop at a time and watch for the bird to swallow before giving more.

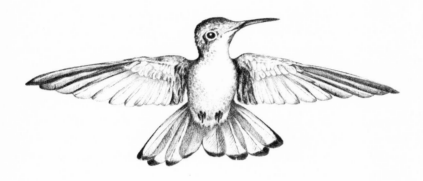

Anna's Hummingbird

These birds need to have food before them at all times. A formula should be made fresh daily with small vials used as feeders so that the food may be replenished frequently. One good place to find such vials is from a florist who carries orchid vials. Any long slender glass vial will do. The nourishing formula can be made with the following ingredients: one ounce of evaporated milk, one ounce of water, half a teaspoon of sugar, two drops of Jeculin (procure at drugstore), one teaspoon of beef broth, and three drops of white syrup. Beef broth can be made by putting a piece of lean raw beef in a tightly covered jar and setting the jar in hot water until the broth is extracted from the beef. This can be made about twice a week and should be kept refrigerated. You may add lean raw beef strained through a garlic press to the formula, but if you do, delete the beef broth. When the bird is able to help himself at the feeder, you should begin to raise fruit flies in the cage by putting peach and/or banana peels in a dish on the bottom of the cage. When the flies emerge they are near enough to be caught by the birds.

The little hummingbird loves to sun himself and preen his feathers, and should have a portion of his cage in the sun. Caution must be taken to leave a shaded area where he may move out of the direct sun. This is true for all caged birds and animals.

The wings of the hummingbird are fastened to the body in such a manner that they give a rotary motion, permitting the bird to hover, fly backward or dash forward. The wings beat at a terrific speed, probably fifty to seventy beats per second. In migration these birds can make a nonstop flight of almost five hundred miles.

Unfortunately, hummingbirds are being decimated by the extensive use of pesticides. The insects on which they thrive and the flowers from which they obtain their nectar are constantly barraged with sprays by those who are either unaware of or unconcerned with the destruction these poisons wreak upon wildlife.

Chapter 2

CARE OF THE FURRED

BABY ANIMALS

Requirements for animal care differ somewhat with each species. As in the bird section, I will attempt to simplify the procedures to cover as many little creatures as possible.

Baby opossums found clinging to the mother or in her pouch after she has been killed or injured need help. Normally they stay with the mother for about a year, clinging to her back for long periods of time. These little fellows are hard to raise, but it can be done. Do not be surprised if they eat one another; although not common, such cannibalism may occur.

On the other hand, baby skunks, raccoons, rabbits and other little animals which are old enough to follow after mother quite often are better off left alone to fend for themselves. This does not include the venturesome kind that have fallen from the nest too soon, eyes still unopened and obviously in need of nursing.

Sick animals are not often found: nature has a way of taking care of this situation with predators. If they are sick enough to be able to be picked up by humans, they are quite often beyond recovery. The kindest thing to do in this case—and this includes the many little birds one finds, particularly in the fall—is to make them comfortable. Provide food and water and privacy from curious humans, and hope for the best. If the creature is badly injured, contact your local SPCA, Animal Rescue League, or a veterinarian and have it mercifully put to sleep. A relationship with these groups should be established and nurtured as often expert help will be needed to aid in the treatment of an injured wildling.

Wildlife experts and zoologists agree that there is usually little danger from rabies or other wild animal diseases. However, reasonable precautions should be taken to guard against scratches, cuts or bites. In some areas, foxes, skunks, squirrels and other animals have been known to carry rabies. If bitten by a little wild creature you are trying to help, remember he is terrified and it is purely a defensive act. Put yourself in his position and think how you would react if some creature many, many times your size picked you up and handled you! Any animal that has bitten a person should be kept under observation for ten to fifteen days. If it is still healthy at the end of this time it could not have had rabies. I've acquired many a small animal for this very reason. Curious little boys and girls climb trees and put their hands into tree cavities to see if there is anything inside. Certainly mama squirrel will bite; so will the chipmunk; and if it is a skunk in there, well, just bury the clothes and forget it.

We discovered one very good way of removing the skunk odor after battling with it for some time with our two dogs. Canned tomatoes or tomato juice is the only thing that removes the aroma; soap and water just won't work. The base of most perfumes is musk, and musk is the skunk's staunch defense.

Skunks never attack unless in danger and even then they warn you by stamping their front feet while facing you. Once they raise that pretty plume of a tail and whirl around with their back to you . . . leave fast! As long as the tail is down, you are safe. They are very gentle creatures by nature, but will take no nonsense.

I received a phone call one day from a woman who had found a skunk in her window well. She had heard a scrambling sound very early in the morning but didn't investigate until she arose for the day. She didn't want the little fellow hurt, but the "perfume" was quite a deterrent and she wanted to spend the rest of summer in her own home.

I rigged out a long board with burlap tacked on and took off for her house. Sure enough, the skunk had fallen in while investigating some interesting cans and could not climb back out of the steep hole. The plank was of no interest to him so I had to think of something else. Meanwhile I had cautioned her to stand back. I was really playing this one by ear—I had been talking softly and gently to the little fellow so that by then he was completely unafraid of me. I could even reach down and touch his head without alarming him. If I had gone away, he probably would have come out in his own due time, using the board to extricate himself. We couldn't take that chance, though, since it was time for school to be out soon and all we needed then was the clamor of curious, noisy children. I asked if there was any kind of butterfly net, fishing net or such. Fortunately there was on hand an old crabbing net, which is like a butterfly net with long handles and heavy cord netting.

Ever so gently and slowly I slid the net under our young friend and lifted him to the side of the wall. Without a backward look, he headed for the woods on the edge of the property. All three of us breathed a great sigh of relief—two concerned women and one hopefully wiser skunk.

Feeding

Feeding baby wild animals requires knowing just what kind of animal you have. Certainly you would not feed a squirrel raw beef, but you're always safe with warm milk, baby cereal, and eggs—both cooked and raw. (See Feeding Chart.) For the very young who have not yet opened their eyes, the following formula given with an eyedropper or a pet nursing bottle (available at pet shops) will suffice. Never use a glass eyedropper, as their sharp teeth may break it in the mouth. Thoroughly mix together three ounces of homogenized milk (canned milk is too rich), a teaspoon of baby cereal, a drop of corn syrup, about one-fourth teaspoon of calcium gluconate, one drop of vitamin oil (Viosteral or any good baby vitamin oil will do), a few drops of wheat germ oil, and one-half teaspoon of Esbilac, which may be found at a veterinary office or drugstore. Keep this mixture refrigerated until ready for use, and then warm to body temperature by setting the filled bottle in warm water before feeding. Be very careful not to make it too hot, and also be sure that the milk is fresh and has not soured. Infant animals won't take soured milk. Check the bottle to make sure that the flow is not too fast or the opening so small that no formula gets to the animal. Plastic medicine droppers can also be used. Milk bubbling out of the nostrils is an indication that the animal is getting too much at once. You may even have to burp the little creature occasionally.

Chipmunks, mice, rabbits, squirrels and other rodents are seed and nut eaters and in time you should start offering them peanuts, nuts, lettuce and such. I have also found that they are very fond of applesauce and grapes. Young skunks, opossums, foxes and other meat eaters should be offered lean ground beef, fish, fruits, eggs and some table scraps. Never give them ham or pork, which are the hardest meats of all to digest. These foods should be offered when they start to get active, exploring their cage with eyes wide open. Canned tuna and salmon are also liked by some animals.

Feed a nursing fawn on milk, with the addition of Pablum and vitamins and Esbilac to the milk. House the animal in a shed with an outside run that has grass and undergrowth, and supply it with water. Bedding for the stall should be straw and hay. When hunting season comes in the fall, keep the young deer confined to his quarters for safety. There are deer on our property and I keep salt blocks along the edge of the tree line and in the small orchard, where the deer have a ball with the apples. Deer are easy to handle here, but not everyone lives where the natural habitat of the deer is so readily accessible.

When the mating instinct and the need to be wild gain control of the animal's behavior, then it is time to sever its relations with humans.

Treat starving creatures the same as you would those which are in shock or unconscious. Feed them something easy to ingest and digest, like warm milk, which provides nourishment and the moisture necessary to alleviate dehydration. If the animal is unconscious, turn the head sideways so that the milk can run over the tongue and out in case the animal cannot swallow. Allow them warmth and quiet.

Last summer I found an apparently dead raccoon on the highway. Its eyes and mouth were filled with sand from its struggles, and it was unconscious. I poured water into the eyes and through the mouth while the animal was on its side, to remove the sand. After the tongue was wet and even before all the sand was out of its mouth, the animal was trying to swallow the water. There was no problem with feeding, although the animal was unconscious for about three days. I added raw egg to milk and then tiny bits of bread soaked in milk.

RABBITS

If you are fortunate enough to discover a rabbit's nest in your garden, the best advice is to leave it alone. Leave an area a few feet around the nest untouched and the mother rabbit will continue to take care of her babies. If the young are too small to be out of the nest the chances of successfully raising them are quite doubtful. Just because you do not see the mother rabbit come to the nest does not mean that she isn't caring for her babies. She escaped notice while digging the nest, filling it with soft grass, lining it with fur and giving birth to the babies, so why shouldn't she be just as secretive in taking care of them? Her worst enemies are cats, dogs and especially little humans. It is difficult for children, once they have discovered a nest of any kind, to contain their curiosity. They often keep peeking in and disturbing the nest, with legends of Easter bunnies hopping through their minds.

Stay completely away from the nest and let the mother have a chance to raise her children in peace. Constant turmoil around her home may very well discourage her and cause her to abandon the nest.

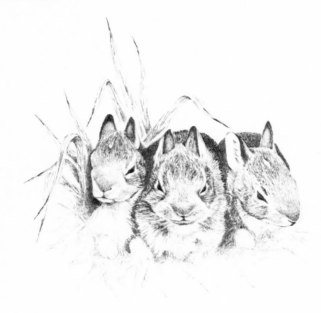

Baby Rabbits

Remember, your chances of successfully raising baby rabbits are doubtful, while the mother rabbit's chances are excellent as long as the nest is not disturbed. If you must watch the nest, do so from inside the house and do it quietly so she will not see your movements at a window or door. She will slip in and nurse, re-cover the nest and leave as quietly as she came. However, she will not be far away, always on guard and ready to try to lure an intruding predator away from the nest. Rabbits, because of their coloring, ability to sit absolutely motionless, speed and erratic movements, are well able to cope with their natural enemies.

Young rabbits grow very rapidly. When they are still tiny enough to sit comfortably in the palm of your hand they will be making little forages away from the nest to eat clover and grass. They are very swift and can squeeze their tiny, pliable bodies through an almost impossibly small opening.

Confine your cat or dog to give the rabbits time to mature and leave the nest. As more and more of their natural habitat is developed, the animals become surrounded by buildings and are forced to nest wherever they can find a relatively quiet and unmolested place.

I have found that by putting a foot-high piece of chicken wire around the edges of bulb beds I can protect my flowers from rabbits and other trespassers. A foot-high picket fence is equally effective; either is easily set up and removed when no longer needed. If you feel that rabbits are a nuisance around your yard, trap them in a humane manner and take them to open country for release, where they will have a much better chance for survival.

However, if you do get the job of mothering a nest of rabbits (I especially remember the five presented to me one Easter morning), here are a few tips for their care.

Tiny rabbits may be fed three ounces of homogenized milk to which has been added a teaspoon of mixed baby cereal. Let the mixture stand until dissolved. Keep the formula refrigerated in a tightly covered jar. Heat for feeding by setting the jar in a pan of warm water, do not overheat. Give five feedings per day at intervals of three hours. Feeding at night is not necessary.

Keep the rabbits warm and dry. House them in a box long enough to let just the end which contains the bedding sit on top of the incubator. Be sure the sides of the box are high enough to keep them from jumping or falling out. A window screen across the top allows for ventilation and checks any sudden forceful jumps. Rabbits can jump incredible distances and move so fast that it is easy to lose them.

For bedding use a small box filled with facial tissue, placed in the larger box. The end which is off the incubator is the place to put food once they start feeding themselves. A small shallow container is needed for water. When they are large enough to get their own food, supply the rabbits with bread and the usual formula along with pieces of apple and grain. They need fresh clover and grass twice a day, and be sure to leave them a fresh bunch at bedtime. Also be sure that the area where you get their grasses is free of any pesticides or weed killers. Most likely they will be toxic to baby rabbits.

Little rabbits need to be put outside at an early age. A weather-protected wire cage with a wire bottom is fine. If using a bird cage, be sure to check the holes where the feeding dishes fit. These little animals can get out of anything they can get their heads through, and their heads aren't as large as they seem to be. The wire bottom should be made of one-inch mesh wire to allow them to nibble on the grass. Move the cage frequently for cleanliness and to provide a fresh supply of grass. Keep water in the cage with the apples, carrots, grain, bread and milk.

As soon as you feel that the rabbits can forage for themselves, take them to the country for release. Select an area where they are away from the highway. A thickly grown hedgerow at the edge of a pasture or field is ideal for both protection and food. A young rabbit four inches in length in his natural sitting position is well able to forage for himself and should not be kept in captivity any longer. Jack rabbits are considerably larger so the baby should be about the size of a full grown cottontail before being released.

SQUIRRELS

Squirrels, even those too young to have fur, are (unlike rabbits) fairly easy to raise if you follow a few sensible rules. First be sure that the squirrel is really in need of raising. Many of them fall out of trees, but if left alone, the mother will come right down and take the baby by the scruff of the neck back to the nest.

Artificial heat for the very young, always a necessity, should be provided by a homemade incubator. An even temperature is essential, as are regular feeding habits and a minimum of handling.

Raising a squirrel from infancy falls into three phases: birth to four weeks; four weeks to two months; two months to release time. The treatment, housing and feeding will vary during this time. A squirrel's eyes usually open between the nineteenth and twenty-first day, so you will be able to judge his age by this.

Use a medicine dropper to feed very tiny squirrels, regulating the flow of milk. Again, never use a glass eyedropper. Little squirrels are usually quite greedy and sometimes choke themselves in their eagerness to satisfy hunger. By feeding on a bath towel on a table, you will have better control of the animal and the flow of milk. Never leave an animal unattended on a table; it may scramble about and fall to the floor.

Use the following formula for the best results: to three ounces of homogenized milk, add one teaspoonful of mixed baby cereal. Let stand until dissolved, then add about four drops of white corn syrup or half a teaspoonful of Esbilac. Start infants out on this mixture, or feed them just milk and baby cereal at first, adding the Esbilac after a few days. Esbilac, obtainable from drugstores or veterinarians, contains many nutrients young animals need to develop properly.

Make a fresh formula each day, keep tightly covered and refrigerated. Heat at each feeding to body temperature.

Wash the medicine dropper after each feeding. Milk sours

very quickly and if the animal takes any soured milk, which is uncommon, it could cause illness. Often if it is sour or too hot, they will not accept it again.

A baby squirrel raised in captivity can be very susceptible to colds. Never bathe the animal. Do not use cedar shavings sold in local pet shops for hamster and mouse cages as they may cause a coating of cedar dust to settle on the animal, clogging the nostrils and causing discomfort. If it is necessary to clean him, use tissues with a bit of baby oil or white petroleum jelly. Never use cotton. Cotton may leave moisture, adding to the danger of pneumonia.

During the time he is learning to eat by himself, the squirrel will get formula on his feet and face. Clean off large spills with a washcloth and warm water before you put him back in his bed.

Use a cardboard box with sides twelve inches high for infant squirrels. An old fish tank is ideal, provided you cover the top with a mesh lid to keep them from scrambling out. It prevents drafts and gives them a safe temporary home. Fit the box into the incubator, and use facial tissue for bedding: it is easily disposed of for cleanliness, is lightweight, and absorbs heat. Little squirrels will burrow under tissue for warmth and can readily crawl on top for a cooler temperature. Enough warmth will come through the bottom of the carton to keep them comfortable. As soon as each little squirrel is fed return him immediately to bed. He will sleep through to the next feeding. Never let newspaper come in direct contact with the animals, as the lead in the printing ink makes them ill.

After infancy, when the squirrel's eyes have been open for about a week, it is time to start training him to eat formula from a dish. Use a can or jar lid about three inches in diameter and not over an inch deep for a feeding dish. Do not feed the animal in his bed—use an extra cardboard carton as a feeding room. He will be quite messy at first and the feeding room will

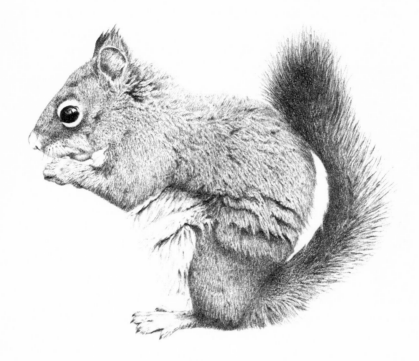

Red Squirrel

prevent the bed from getting soiled. Use paper on the bottom
of the box.

Line the bottom of the feed dish with a piece of white bread,
then pour enough formula over it to make it quite moist. Gently
put the animal's mouth against the food. You may have to do
this several times until he learns to suck on the bread. Some
learn very fast, others require a good deal of patience. In my
childhood we weaned calves to drink out of a pail by the same
procedure: a calf's nose was put in the pail of milk, and once
a taste of it got on his tongue, we had it made.

Alternate the feedings, by hand and from the dish, so that feeding habits are not changed too suddenly. As soon as the squirrel eats readily from the dish, drop the hand-feeding. Lining the dish with bread will prevent the animal from getting too much milk in his nose and choking. Only attempt to feed one squirrel at a time. Until they get adept at it, they leave the food, walk through it and in general get themselves and the whole box into a mess. The baby may look rather revolting for awhile, but ignore it. As soon as he indicates that he has had enough food, put him back in his warm bed to dry out. If he is drippy with milk, use a dry terrycloth towel to gently remove some of the debris. Do not attempt to bathe him; it is better to have him dirty than dead from a sudden cold. When he has grown enough to give up the incubator he will need a variety of other foods in addition to bread and milk.

The diet required is quite simple. Here we have a nut, fruit, and salad eater. If you don't believe the salad part, just keep an eye on next year's crop of crocus, tulips and daffodils—the flowers, not the bulbs. They are mostly herbivorous; however, as in all cases, there are some exceptions to every rule. Weevil fragments found regularly in gray squirrel stomachs are probably ingested accidently with acorns. Certain insect foods, like caterpillars and cocoons, beetles and ants, are occasionally eaten. Some individuals eat birds' eggs and even nestlings on occasion.

A large cage is needed for a young squirrel to climb and exercise in, at least three feet wide by four feet in height. However, on occasion a large dog-carrying cage has worked very well when there are no more than one or two babies. Lengths of tree limb large enough to afford good climbing should be fastened in the cage. For bedding use a bag of some woolen material like an old blanket. Hang the bag in one corner of the cage, securing the top to two sides of the cage so that the top will be held partially open. Put about a dozen tissues in the bottom of the bag. You may have to show the animals how to get into the bag at first, but soon they will learn to climb the wire sides of the cage and get down into the bed. By hanging the bed well off the floor, the paper on the floor may be more readily removed when cleaning the cage. Secure a small container for water to the side of the cage so they cannot tip it over.

At this stage extra food is needed. Supply them twice a day with bread and milk, and also give small pieces of apple, shelled pecans and walnuts, peanuts and sunflower seeds. Chicken scratch, which contains corn and wheat, is an excellent addition. You will have a great deal of fun watching their first attempts to hold a nut to eat. From now on, it is much easier to care for them.

At two months of age the squirrel should be starting to acclimate for release. He needs to be kept outside, but protected from marauders and predators. He should be able to get onto the ground, climb trees and generally develop the skills he will need to care for himself. If your yard is free of dogs and cats his new freedom won't be much of a problem. However, having been hand-raised he will be less wary of danger than any wild animal should be. He still needs to be watched and fed, and his cage closed at night for protection. A nail keg (if you can find one these days) with a weatherproof top on it will do very nicely as a bed. The bag should be placed in the keg as bedding since it is a familiar thing and means home to the animal. Some measure of freedom during the day and confinement at night is the best policy. A box house could be erected in a favorite tree, but be sure it is placed in a position a wandering cat cannot reach, and make the opening large enough for only the squirrel.

Never keep a squirrel or any creature confined longer than necessary. If you acquire an animal late in the fall you should house him through the cold months of winter since he hasn't had the time or the know-how to make a home or lay in a food supply by release time. If it is a spring baby, release it early in the summer so it will have a chance to learn to care for itself before the start of cold weather. Squirrels have babies as late as November and as early as February.

Use caution and common sense when feeding a squirrel that is old enough to release. Do not hand food to a squirrel, but drop it and let him pick it up. Although he might not mean to, he might nip your finger in his eagerness to get the food. I have had them take peanuts out of my hand with the greatest delicacy, and on the other hand, I have, in my carelessness, been severely bitten by my little charges. Play it safe. With their razor-sharp teeth, suitable for chiseling nuts and bark, the bite can be very deep and painful. I still have a deadened nerve on the end of my thumb from a squirrel bite. This happened not from trying to feed it, but from giving it badly needed medication. It was my own fault in handling, and even though I was wearing heavy veterinarian gloves, the bite went through the fabric. So take care!

Flying squirrels are nocturnal animals. When released they do not build an open nest, as do gray and red squirrels, but nest instead in a cavity of a tree. They will also use a bird house if one is provided. The opening in a tree house for either flying or red squirrels should be much smaller than for larger varieties.

It is advisable to separate the male squirrels from the females when they are still tiny and on the bottle, especially if you have several to raise. In their quest for food while in bed, the females often mistake a portion of the males' anatomy for their missing mother's teats. After they are old enough to feed themselves, they can be put in a nest together, but prior to that keep them separated.

RACCOONS

I adore these beautiful, friendly, intelligent animals. They must be smart to have survived as well as they have with the odds so much against them. Hunters, dogs, cars, poison bait, and loss of woodlands have taken a heavy toll of wild raccoons.

Raccoons are nocturnal animals, sleeping through the day in a hollow tree and roaming for food and adventure during the night. They live in every one of the continental forty-nine states. The name raccoon comes from an Algonquin Indian word, *arakun,* meaning "he scratches with his hands." He resembles a little bear, especially when he waddles along the ground and sits up begging for food, or stands on his hind legs. He has the most beautiful and sensitive "hands" in the animal kingdom. He also has some bad habits, by human standards, which cause him to be termed a "varmint," hunted continuously. He eats almost anything: bird eggs, baby birds, chickens; and he can have a real ball in a corn field. Fruits, especially grapes, make him persona non grata to many a farmer.

One little one I raised vividly impressed me. How this baby raccoon managed to land unharmed at the base of a large oak tree and live is still a mystery to me, but there he was, six days old, totally blind, and very unhappy and hungry. Perhaps the mother raccoon moved her brood and had lost this one in the process. Or, perhaps he was clinging to her as she descended the tree, lost his hold and tumbled to the ground. The mother must have been frightened off by an unusual noise, because normally she would have gone down and brought him back up the tree.

A little girl found him and her father rode miles on a motor scooter to deliver him to me for care. From the very first he was an adventurous little fellow and very vocal when hungry. With his growl and personality it was natural to call him Tiger. He greedily took his first meal from a medicine dropper, and then settled down in the corner of a box on a bath towel. Like most furry babies, he only stayed awake long enough to eat, and slept the remainder of the time. He didn't seem to mind his change in hours and habits. He was fed and slept alternately during the day and seemed to sleep quite soundly the whole night through after an evening feeding at ten o'clock.

I found him to be a very clean little animal, as have been all the raccoons I've raised. From the very first, although he was still blind, he knew where his bed was and never soiled it, seeming instinctively to distinguish between the end of the box furnished for soiling purposes and the bath towels provided for his bed. He didn't seem to mind either that his quarters weren't that fancy, merely a long pasteboard carton (the kind used to ship bananas in), or that he was lodged on the floor. The sides of his box were about fourteen inches high and provided safety from falls as well as a shield from drafts.

Tiger seemed to thrive immediately on a diet of homogenized milk, and was such a little pig that I only fed him from a medicine dropper a few times before providing him with a baby bottle. Within a few days I began to add a level teaspoon of Esbilac. In about sixteen days his eyes were open and he had his first look at the world.

At about the same time his eyes opened he also learned that he could reach the top of the box by stretching up against its sides. In this way he also learned to climb over it; he thought this was great fun, and climbed in and out at will. I provided an old woolen sweater as an outside bed, wedged between the wall and the box, and he took many naps on the sweater. Sometimes he would take a little walk around the dinette, but he never seemed to stray far from his quarters. If startled by something he would head for his box and scramble over the side into his bed. He still remained very clean in his habits and never soiled the floor, a trait I have found in other raccoons I have raised. Unlike puppies and cats, raccoons housebreak themselves.

Needless to say he was the center of attention. The problem confronting me was to love him and give him plenty of attention without spoiling him. Each person who raises a wildling must face this problem if he is not to be making pets out of creatures who rightfully belong in the wild.

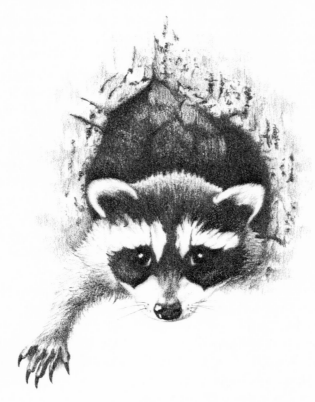

Raccoon

As soon as Tiger was able to eat the formula poured over bread in a saucer, instead of from a bottle, I began to let him have some freedom in an unoccupied outdoor aviary. He loved this, climbing the wire sides and exploring every inch of space.

His diet was increased to include hard-boiled eggs, grapes, and pieces of chicken. He also loved crisp bacon and, of all things, marshmallows. Although at first we brought him into the house at night, it was only a few days before I decided to move his bed outside. I used the same bedding he was accustomed to and placed it high up in the aviary in a wooden box nailed to a shelf. I secured a length of tree limb about eight feet long and six inches across to the shelf, leaving one end on the ground. This provided a very handy stairway to his bed and on it he learned to climb. He was quite clumsy, losing his hold on the limb and running into things in his efforts to play. I often wondered if he would ever be able to take care of himself.

Tiger was in the house off and on during the day, and was allowed to roam around freely. He was never destructive, however, and in this he was an exception to the rule. I wouldn't advise this freedom once a raccoon reaches a few months of age. (Two other little raccoons, in only five minutes, spilled black ceramic paint on a table and left beautiful little handprints all over a red sofa. It really looked great—instant block printing.)

If Tiger decided to investigate a trashcan and was scolded, he would head for the safety of the small space between the refrigerator and the wall and peer out until he decided that all was friendly again and it was safe to venture forth. He seemed to know his family and was very wary of strangers. He associated me with his source of food and my daughter with playtime. She would sit on the floor and roughhouse with him by the hour. He would hide under the skirts of a wingback chair, dive out at her and really have a good old tumbling skirmish.

He also loved to get on the back of a sofa and remove combs and pins from my daughter's hair and run off with them. He enjoyed being taken to the creek that flows in front of our home. He would wade around the edge of the water, feeling in the sand with his little hands for small stones which he would wash thoroughly. He refused to stay there by himself, and always followed us back to the house. I kept a large pan of water in his cage and he would gather up pebbles and wash them in the water.

A common statement made about raccoons is that they always wash their food before eating it. I have found the raccoon to be more of a "feeler" or "dunker" than a "washer." Frequently grapes and chicken are eaten without the benefit of scrubbing in the water pan. It has also been claimed that the animal has no salivary glands and washes its food to help in swallowing. Both of these theories have been disproved in studies of animal habits and physiognomy.

Much of the food gathered by raccoons in the wild is secured by the banks of creeks and ponds as well as in the water. Fish, crayfish, frogs and mussels, tadpoles and minnows are greatly enjoyed. They love grapes and apples. Garbage cans are another source of tidbits, more so now as their natural sources of food are supplanted by housing developments. They eat not only meat and fruit, but insects, berries, grubs and grain.

Raccoons are very curious creatures and get into everything. One little female raccoon had the habit of plunging her hands in a bucket of water I kept beside the house. One day a bucket of paint was left on the ground and in went both paws. A more disgusted animal you never saw. She took off for the stream and scrubbed and scrubbed, uttering all the while the chirping, rasping, piercing scream that raccoons use when frightened or angry. She suffered no ill effects, but her water bucket days were over. She never repeated the performance.

We released Tiger in our back yard, into an area where there is an open window well. There isn't a basement under the house, so he had the whole subfloor area for protection from weather and harm. He still lives there, with a little female raccoon I later released. She is still quite tame and allows me to approach and touch her, but Tiger has reverted to the wild as he should, and disappears under the house if approached. I needn't have worried about his environment; he had help when he really needed it, was released very gradually into a safe place, and was left to reacclimate to his natural way of living. I still feed both raccoons every evening in a bucket wedged between two cinder blocks so that it cannot be tipped over, protected from the weather by a plastic screen. I often see the animals eating from their supply of giblets, bread and milk, hard-boiled or raw egg mixed with milk and bread, grapes, and of course, their daily treat of marshmallows.

I often hear them playing under the house, and sometimes racing across the roof, which they reach by climbing the telephone pole directly beside the kitchen. I will definitely capture and take these little animals when we move in the near future. I fear that the next tenants of the house might not have the same interest in preserving such active wild friends.

I had not given much thought to raccoons until I raised Tiger. He was such a delightful animal, and so responsive to kindness; yet he was all male animal, and wild, and needed to be returned to the wild as he came of age. His reorientation was so gradual that he didn't miss us, since his food was there for the taking. He was sheltered without being confined and could still see his "family" when the notion suited him. This gradual release is necessary to the well-being of all wild creatures which have been raised by humans. It is a great responsibility, one not to be taken lightly. Help the animals without being selfish: don't keep them too long. Release them in a safe area.

Raccoons remain in their natural family for almost a year, and to Tiger we were family. By simply being friendly, inviting him to come into the house for a romp now and then, and providing food and shelter without confining him to a cage, I was able to enjoy him while he was growing into a beautiful and self-sufficient animal. He didn't trust our dog and I never encouraged a friendship between the two: it seemed safer for him to remain wary of any potential enemy.

The exploitation of these animals in pet shops is appalling. They really do not make good pets, and after a year they get restive and revert to the wild state. They hate being picked up at this time and will bite if need be to let you know they want friendship on their terms, not yours. They are very independent animals. If you have the land and trees to warrant it, they will stay in your area and come to you for handouts from time to time, but they won't cuddle after a year's time, so don't attempt it.

DEER

If you ever inherit a fawn to raise and have not had this wonderful experience before, here are a few tips for making the work easy for you and pleasant for the fawn. If your yard is not fenced, do fence in an area at least fifty feet square. This will give the animal room to exercise. Use steel posts, which are easy to install and remove when they are no longer needed. Six-food-wide chicken wire is also practical and easy to install. Try to put the fenced area around a tree or shrubs that you do not mind having pruned a bit. As the fawn grows and begins to nibble on green leaves, he may denude the lower branches.

Three four-by-eight sheets of exterior plyboard will make a great house. Use two pieces of the plywood as an end and a side. Make the other end and remaining side of chicken wire, using a post to support the wire and corner of the roof. A two-by-four is fine for this post. Put the remaining piece of plywood on top and place roofing paper over that to shed water. With the inclusion of a small doorway, you have a finished barn for the fawn. I like having a door to shut the fawn in at night while it is quite small, just for safety, and for my own peace of mind. Fresh water must always be available, a small block of salt also.

Food is no problem. To homogenized cow's milk add four tablespoons of mixed Pablum cereal and a tablespoon of Esbilac.

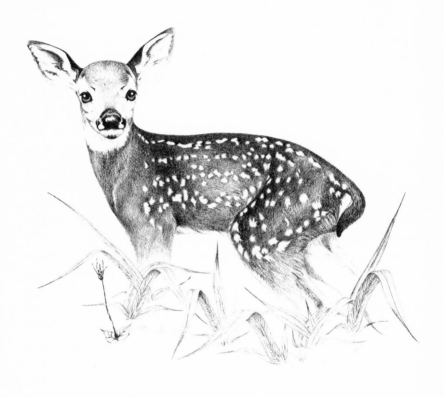

Fawn

Use a sixteen-ounce bottle such as a discarded brandy bottle upon which a lamb's nipple (procure at drugstore) will fit. Set the bottle in hot water until the formula is just warm. Give five daily feedings and decrease these gradually as the fawn begins to nibble grass and leaves and shows an interest in grain offered; intermediate chicken scratch is fine. At about this time you could offer the formula in a pan, poured over a slice of wholewheat bread. He will suck the bread and soon learn to take all feedings in this manner. If flies are becoming a problem for your charge you may place dark bamboo curtains over the wire on the house, affording a dark area where the fawn can get away from the flies. I use a very mild fly spray (the kind used for horses) to rub the fawn's coat to repel flies. Expert advice about sprays, medications, etc., is always useful and may save you considerable trouble. These little animals become very tame and will follow after you as does a dog. They love having little special treats such as carrots, apples, shelled peanuts and marshmallows. The animal will be fortunate if your area is rural and free of dogs, so that when release time comes he can readily acclimate to his natural environment. If there are other deer in the area he will find them. Sometimes a fawn will develop a diarrhea, probably the result of a change of diet. Do not attempt to treat the animal with home or drugstore remedies. Your veterinarian will be able to prescribe a proper medicine and dosage.

I would not advise keeping a fawn in captivity much over six months. It may be against the law in your state to keep these animals confined in any way. In fact, most states require permits for keeping any wild animals or birds. I have a female raccoon now that was shipped from Louisiana to two young boys who lived in an apartment near me. No attempt was made to determine if there were adequate facilities for the animal or whether the boys could keep it in the area without a permit. The animal lost two front toes from improper caging in shipment, and was hurt and frightened when it arrived. Moreover, it had outgrown its collar and would have strangled in a short time. It bit one of the boys and was quarantined here where it will remain until spring, when I will release it on our farm. I am sure that it will hate humans for the rest of its life.

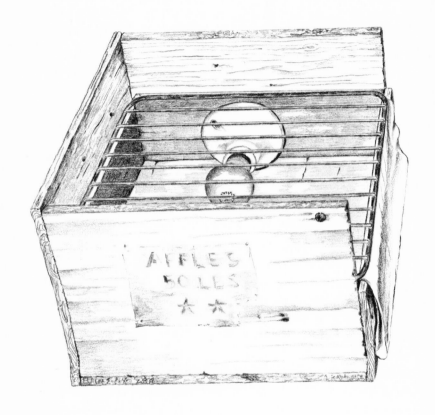

Incubator

Chapter 3

SPECIAL EQUIPMENT

INCUBATORS

A great help in raising baby birds or animals is the homemade incubator. The cost is under a dollar, the benefits are invaluable. Its constant temperature substitutes for the warmth of nest and parents better than any other method.

The incubator is very easy to construct. All that is needed is a wooden box about a foot high and at least fourteen inches square, an ordinary light bulb fixture, and enough electric cord to reach the outlet or wall plug. Secure the fixture near the bottom, over the hole which you have drilled for the electric cord. Nail four pieces of wooden molding around the inside of the box just above the light fixture. Set a discarded grate from an ice box or an oversized cake rack on top of the molding; or place a couple of crossbars as supports and use a piece of hardware cloth instead of a grate. This size incubator will house nine plastic berry boxes which may be used as nests for tiny birds.

When using this versatile device for mammals, keep them in a cardboard carton with one end on the incubator. Drop about two dozen facial tissues lightly over the babies. They can then crawl under the tissues for warmth at the bottom of the box. Do the same with the plastic berry box nests for birds. The box is kept at a steady temperature by the light bulb, and if it gets too warm the little animals can easily climb on top of the tissues for a cooler temperature. Facial tissues are easily removed for cleanliness, and are kept dry by the steady heat from the bulb.

As mentioned previously, do not use grass cuttings for bedding since it is damp and cold against the animals' bodies; and, in caring for any kind of baby animal which chews, do not use newspaper on the bottom of the cage because the ink, made with lead, may poison them. Use a 25-watt bulb to provide just enough heat and not too much. But do not leave an unshaded light bulb burning near an animal or bird so that they are forced to look at it. Light stress will decrease their ability to heal or relax. Keep the incubator in a room as warm as the one you live in. Never keep animals in a cold room or a damp basement or garage. If possible the animals should be kept in a room in which a minimum of activity takes place, once again so as not to stress them with noise and vibrations. The incubator should be at 85°, use an outdoor thermometer to be sure.

When the animals have grown larger and have begun climbing or jumping over the sides of the cardboard carton, transfer them to a bird cage in which you have provided tissues for bedding. Set the cage on the incubator. Animals will not be able to get out and their warmth will not be disrupted. Remove artificial heat as soon as the wildlings are old enough to do without it, after their eyes have been open for about a week.

In an emergency, temporary incubators can be made of three-pound coffee tins with plastic tops. Punch holes in a can so that plenty of air gets in, line the bottom with many layers of tissue, and place the can on a heating pad set at low. One does not always have everything on hand when the occasion arises and it is very important to provide warmth as soon as possible. Injured creatures need warmth as much as lost young'uns. Warmth and quiet are prerequisites for healing as well as natural growth in captivity.

CAGES AND PENS

Once small birds and animals become dissatisfied with being kept in a nest, they need to be treated differently. At this point in their growth they need the addition of different foods to their diet. They also need to be outside in larger quarters so that they may begin to adjust to the elements which they will encounter when released. They need to become accustomed to outdoor sounds and the voices of others of their own kind, and to learn the sounds of warning given by others when danger is near. This is the first step in their rehabilitation back to the wild. They need perches placed at different levels for exercise, and the sun above and the ground below to move about on if they are to become healthy and strong. For this they need an outside cage or aviary which is protected from predators so that they can move about freely while learning to care for themselves.

I prefer a small outside pen completely covered with wire netting, with one end sheltered and a roof over all. The sheltered end contains two boxes, both with perches, one at ground level and one at roof level. Leave the front open on the lower box to shelter those who are not yet able to get up onto the higher perches. The upper box may be divided into two compartments with a door on each. This serves as a night shelter for birds.

Young birds should not be left to fly around in aviaries at night. A predator climbing over the cage at night will frighten the birds, who may fly against the wire and injure themselves. A lovely young wood thrush was found one morning with a broken leg after being left in an inadequately protected cage. Her injuries were mostly internal; she did not recover from the experience. At dusk birds should be placed in the upper boxes and the doors closed for the night. If the weather is cold, a curtain of cloth, plastic, or even newspaper may be placed over the front of the box to afford extra protection. Newspapers in the bottoms of the boxes for such maturing, non-nibbling creatures will insure cleanliness and should be changed daily.

I have found that a four-foot-by-six-foot pen about six feet high is the most practical aviary. Make a frame of two-by-fours to set the aviary on. Secure a heavy, fine wire mesh to the bottom of the frame, and fill the frame half full with clean dirt and sand. The aviary corner supports and roof, made the same width and length as the bottom frame, may then be secured on top of the frame. This eliminates the ever present danger of predators digging into the aviary from the bottom. The dirt may be removed and replaced from time to time. The aviary may be made in sections, with the top, ends, and sides separate so that they may be knocked down for easy storage or moving. I have used inch mesh chicken wire but, though it is more expensive, half-inch mesh hardware cloth or stucco netting is the most practical in the long run. In using chicken wire there is the danger of strangulation for small birds. The hardware cloth is smaller, affords more protection, and will not rust. Strips of tin may be used on the sides and back to make the sheltered end of the aviary. I have also used tin on top and secured roofing paper over that.

If I seem to dwell on the use of these pens for birds, it is because you will probably wind up with more birds than animals. The cage can be used equally well for raccoons and squirrels. Obviously you don't need such elaborate preparations for ground animals like rabbits and skunks.

This size pen has many advantages. While it affords small birds enough wing space for exercise, it is still small enough to allow reaching the young who are still being hand-fed. I have found that all I need to do is enter the pen, kneel down, and remain in that position to feed. The little ones cluster around and beg for their food with much fluttering of wings and vocal supplication. Even those who are picking up food for themselves get into the act. Some of the youngest and most timid may remain in a corner of the pen and yell for their food, and it may take a few days before they learn to approach for feeding. It is easy to reach these birds in a pen this size. It is best to remove the youngest from the aviary to a cage in the house at night. If they are much younger or weaker than the other birds, they should not be left in the outside night boxes. They might get trampled by the more aggressive birds. At night I leave out only those birds who can move about readily. It only takes a few days for younger birds to get the feel of the ground and to learn to get up on the perches. By then they are ready to become accustomed to nights outside.

If you find that an aviary detracts from the beauty of your back yard, by all means disguise it as a rose arbor: enough sun will filter through the trellises and vines to satisfy the birds, and the aviary will be most attractive. When unoccupied, small aviaries with the doors left open are nice dry places to feed winter bird visitors.

If you do not care to go into such elaborate preparations, an adequate outside pen can be made for one or two birds by using the frames of large crates. Follow the same procedure used for the larger aviary. These are practical only if you are raising one or two birds, with no thought of future tenants. However, once the neighborhood children find out that there is someone in the area who cares about helping wild creatures, you'll be surprised how many come padding to your door with something for you to help.

Whether you expect to care for only one bird or a dozen, you should arrange for enough equipment to insure the safety and well-being of your visitors. Being so equipped will make your task a pleasure rather than a chore.

Chapter 4

NATURAL WILD DIET
AND
SUGGESTED SUBSTITUTES

These substitutes are suggested to take the place of many foods that a bird or animal normally eats in the wild. Wild foods are difficult to obtain, in many cases impossible. Lettuce, seeds, beef strips and lean ground beef or dog food take the place of many of the grasses, weeds and insects that the bird must have to round out its diet. A balanced diet is every bit as important to them for their well-being as it is to you. Except to such scavengers as the opossum or vulture, *never* give pork in any shape or form. Pork is extremely hard to digest. Night crawlers and worms, though, are usually accepted and not difficult to obtain.

MEAL WORMS

Meal worms are an excellent supplement to the artificial diet. Bluejays, robins, mockingbirds, shrikes and many other insect-eating birds seem to relish a daily feeding of these worms. They are clean, without odor, and very easy to raise.

Use a metal can at least a foot in diameter and a foot high. A large potato chip can, or a small garbage can is excellent. No lid is needed, since the worms cannot climb all the way up the sides of a can. An old washtub or lard can will also work.

Mix together two gallons of bran, the type used to feed farm animals, and about two pounds of cornmeal. Put the mixture in the can. Split open two or three medium potatoes or apples. Either or both may be used. Lay these on top of the meal and bran mixture with the cut side facing down. A piece of worn bath towel, double thickness, is then placed on top of the mixture. A piece of burlap may be used instead of a towel for cover. Almost any pet store can supply you with a few dozen meal worms. Put the worms on top of the bran, cover them, and put them in a moderately cool area of the house and leave them alone. As the worms grow they will crawl up between the two pieces of towel or burlap and may readily be picked up from there. Do not put water on the towel for moisture, as it may mildew. Replenish the supply of apples and/or potatoes every week or so.

The worms develop in three stages: from eggs into worms (they are very tiny at first, but grow to an inch in length); worms into pupas, at which stage they are immobile; and then pupas into black beetles, which in turn lay eggs, starting the cycle again.

I'm sure that a lack of meal worms was responsible for the poor health of many birds brought to me by people who had no knowledge of a proper diet for a wild animal or bird. One blue jay, called Sammy, was as naked as an Easter chick. His feathers refused to grow and the foster parents were at a loss for a reason. Sammy lacked usable protein in his diet since he was fed milk and bread but not the meat he needed in his customary insect diet. I placed him on an accelerated diet of meal worms, ground beef, fruit and hard-boiled eggs, as well as milk and bread. It took a long time on this diet for him to recuperate. He should have been flying when he was brought to me. Finally, his beautiful blue feathers sprouted, and his first flight was a surprise to him and a joy to all of us. Meal worms also helped a cardinal and a loggerhead shrike who were in the same condition.

The dandruff that is always falling from young birds is the flaking off of the sheaths of the feathers. Sometimes birds with dietary deficiencies may pull at their feathers. Be observant of such signs of need—expert advice may be required from a local veterinarian or the Humane Society.

If you are unable to find meal worms at a local pet store, it may be possible to obtain them from granaries or other places where the worms and beetles have established themselves in bran meal or other grains and flours.

Another good source of nutrients is fruit flies. A bowl of decaying fruit, covered with wire or screen, produces fruit flies which can be a source of natural food for some finches, fly-catchers, swallows and hummingbirds, as well as other birds.

That old standby bread and milk is certainly not sufficient in itself and must be added to for proper growth or healing; egg yolk is an excellent food as well. Sweet rolls, doughnuts and such are an added treat for many feathered and furred friends: they like sweets, too. You may come up with successful substitutes of your own. Dog food, dry and moist, has been used to good advantage by many. Supplement this diet in the beginning with vitamins and you're on your way to raising healthy birds and animals.

HOW CHILDREN CAN HELP

With guidance and patience, children can be a great help in raising birds and animals. First, there is the task of gathering foods which are as near to the natural wild food as possible. Second, there is the cleaning of cages and equipment, and third, the feeding cycle itself. Eager-to-help neighborhood children assist in my "zoo" operation. This affords the best opportunity for the study of nature and its relationship to man and his surroundings. It instills a love for the wild, respect for life in its many forms, and a gentleness toward the small and helpless that remains with children through their adult lives.

However, age must be considered in utilizing the services of youngsters. Naturally you would not let most five-year-olds handle a small creature. Each parent will assuredly sense when the child is responsible enough to help. After the bird or animal is well enough to be sent on its way to freedom, let the child stroke it gently while you hold it, explaining why he may not hold it himself. A child has no more wish to be harmful than you, but through his inexperience he could injure the little creature.

Teach older children to care for the creatures the same way you do, and by all means supervise their actions until you are completely sure they can carry on without you. You'll enjoy watching the children develop a real sense of responsibility in caring for wild animals and birds.

Send your would-be assistants out for the berries, seeds, bugs and worms needed for feeding and let them watch you give the food to the birds. Show them how to clean out the cages without frightening the inhabitants, and explain each thing you do.

Suggest that they look up the bird or animal in library books and tell you what they find. Where do birds go when they migrate? Is it a migratory bird? Does a certain animal hibernate in the winter? What benefit is it to mankind? How has mankind affected it? What are its habits? Do the children know that the opossum is the oldest living animal in his original prehistoric form? How smart is the raccoon?

You can go on with question after question. In the meantime, you are getting help raising your charges, while educating the neighboring youngsters and sensitizing them to life. If you have as much patience with children's questions and exuberance as you have with that baby robin or chipmunk, it will be a joyous experience for all involved.

Food Substitution Chart: Birds

Category	Natural Wild Food	Substitute*
WATER BIRDS		
Loons, Grebes, Water Turkeys	Animal food only: fish, frogs, crabs, aquatic insects	Cod liver oil, bone meal, raw lean beef, fish, frozen herring, night crawlers
Pelicans, Cormorants	Fish, marine worms	Same as above
Swans, Geese	Aquatic vegetation, some grains	Intermediate chicken scratch, wild bird seed, bread, lettuce
Ducks (surface feeding): Mallards, Teals, Pintails, Canvasbacks, Scaups	Vegetation, grasses, wild celery, aquatic animal food, worms	Chicken scratch, bread, grass, lettuce, ground beef, earthworms
Ducks (diving): Sea ducks, Eiders, Harlequins, Old Squaws	Shrimp, mollusks, crabs, small fish	Bread, night crawlers, bone meal, beef, cod liver oil
Gulls and other scavengers	Snails, shrimp, clams, insects, fish	Beef, fish, bread, bone meal, cod liver oil, fish
Terns	Insects, dragonflies, shrimp, small fish	Beef, fish, night crawlers, bread, bone meal, cod liver oil
MARSH AND SHORE BIRDS		
Herons, Egrets, Bitterns, Cranes, Rails, Plovers, Sandpipers, Phalaropes	Crayfish, shrimp, marine worms, frogs, insects, mice, shrews, snails, wild grasses, some grains	Bread, beef strips, night crawlers, lettuce, chicken scratch, bone meal, cod liver oil
UPLAND GAME BIRDS		
Grouse, Doves, Pheasants, Partridges, Pigeons, Turkeys, Bobwhites	Mainly grain, some summer and fall insects	Chicken scratch, wild bird seed, bread
Woodcocks	Mainly earthworms, some grains, flies, beetles, spiders, caterpillars	Earthworms, night crawlers, beef strips, bone meal, cod liver oil

LAND BIRDS

Cuckoos	Mainly tent caterpillars, worms, bugs, grasshoppers	Bone meal, cod liver oil, lean ground beef, beef strips, meal worms, bread
Roadrunners	Snakes, spiders, lizards, grasshoppers, birds	Beef strips, lean ground beef, meal worms, bone meal, cod liver oil
Hummingbirds	Nectar from flowers, tiny insects	Honey, sugar or molasses in water in small vials
Kingbirds, Vireos, Nighthawks, Whippoor-wills, Swifts, Flycatchers, Swallows	Entirely insectivorous, will have to be hand-fed since they catch food in the air	Lean ground beef, very small strips of raw beef, bread and milk, meal worms
Kingfishers	Fish, minnows, crabs, frogs, locust, lizards	Fish, beef strips, night crawlers
Woodpeckers, Flickers, Sapsuckers	Grubs, ants, bores, beetles, berries in the winter	Meal worms, bread and milk, beef strips, suet, ground beef
Larks	Seeds, grasshoppers, beetles, caterpillars	Meal worms, wild bird seed, bread
Magpies, Crows, Ravens (Carrion eaters and scavengers)	Insects, acorns, fruit, small birds	Ground beef, beef, chicken scratch, bread, hard-boiled egg, bone meal, cod liver oil
Jays	Large insects, some frogs, mice, acorns and sunflower seeds	Ground beef, hard-boiled egg, sunflower seeds, peanuts, nuts
Chats, Chickadees, Titmice, Nuthatches, Towhees	Pine seeds, sunflower seeds, acorns, poison ivy, beetles, weevils, ants, other insects	Shelled peanuts, nuts, blueberries, apples, wild bird seed, sunflower seeds, suet
Mockingbirds, Starlings, Brown Thrashers, Warblers, Robins, Thrushes, Catbirds, Bluebirds, Cedar Waxwings	Holly, grapes, cherries, sumac, pokeweed, Virginia creeper, cedar pyracantha, worms, ants, beetles. Fruits in fall and winter	Apples, raisins, sour cherries, bread, suet, ground beef, meal worms, earthworms
Cowbirds, Sparrows, Blackbirds, Meadowlarks	Crickets, insects, weed seeds	Wild bird seed, scratch, bread, suet, ground beef
Orioles, Tanagers	Caterpillars, ants, spiders, wild fruits	Apples, cherries, blueberries, bread, ground beef, meal worms, suet

Grosbeaks, Purple Finches, Cardinals, Buntings, Crossbills	Insects, bugs, beetles, sunflower seeds, dogwood, sumac, tree buds, fruits	Meal worms, suet, sunflower seeds, cherries, wild bird seed, bread
Shrikes	Grasshoppers, beetles, caterpillars, wasps, small rodents, frogs	Meal worms, ground beef, shrimp, chicken, bread, lettuce, baby mice

PREDATORS

Hawks: Red-tailed, Cooper's	Mice, rats, rodents of all kinds, birds	Lean strips of beef, mice, milk, chicken, bone meal, cod liver oil
Sparrow Hawks (Kestrels)	Grasshoppers, insects, wasps, locusts, very occasionally, small birds	Beef strips, meal worms, milk, grasshoppers, bone meal, mice
Ospreys (Fish Hawks)	Fish	Fish, beef strips, chicken
Kites	Lizards, snakes, frogs, grasshoppers, snails	Shrimp, beef, fish, chicken, mice
Bald Eagles	Fish, rodents, ducks, birds	Fish, lean beef, bone meal, cod liver oil, mice
Golden Eagles	Rodents, birds	Beef chunks, chicken, mice, bone meal
Large Owls	Rodents of all kinds	Milk, beef, mice, rats, chicken, bone meal, cod liver oil
Elf, Pigmy Owls	Large insects, moths, beetles	Meal worms, grasshoppers, moths, beetles, beef strips, ground beef

*Moistened kibbled dogfood is preferable to beef in most cases.

Food Substitution Chart: Animals

Category	Natural Wild	Food Substitute*
Squirrels, Chipmunks, Mice	Nuts, dogwood, maple buds, oak, acorns, corn, sunflower seeds, fruit	Apples, watermelons, bread, corn, nuts, sunflower seed, chicken scratch, quartered oranges
Rabbits, Woodchucks, Ground Squirrels	Grasses, herbaceous plants, twigs of young trees, corn, oats, clover	Grass, clover, lettuce, apples, carrots, bread, commercial hamster or rabbit food
Opossums	Scavenger — will eat just about anything	Beetles, large insects, grubs, meat, fish, fruit, milk, bread, you name it
Raccoons, Coatimundis, Muskrats, Otters, Minks	Frogs, crayfish, grasshoppers, salamanders, bird eggs, acorns, corn, fruit	Apples, grapes, corn, nuts, bread, large grasshoppers, chicken, ground beef, worms, grubs, beetles, oranges
Skunks	Larval insects, frogs, toads, mice, fruit	Milk, bread, fruits, nuts, meal worms, large grasshoppers, grubs, beetles, ground beef, oranges
Foxes, Coyotes	Mice, rodents, small animals and birds	Beef, grapes, apples, dog food, chicken, oranges
Deer	Vegetarian diet	Grain, wild bird seed, lettuce, carrots, cabbage, corn

*Moistened kibbled dogfood is preferable to beef in most cases.

Chapter 5

TREATMENT FOR INJURIES

METHODS AND TECHNIQUES FOR SPLINTING BIRDS

A bird who depends on flight to escape danger is under great stress when his wings are confined, as is the animal whose ability to escape by running or climbing is curtailed by confinement. However, these creatures will be better able to survive this stress if their treatment is correct: warmth; no sudden movements; seclusion where people are not peeking or poking.

Feed an injured bird or animal and let him rest for awhile before working on his wounds. The only exception is if the wound demands immediate care because of profuse bleeding. In this case the injured might die of stress while his wounds are being treated, but the chances are even greater that he would die by loss of blood; so the risk should be taken. Have on hand a glass of milk containing a little Karo syrup or sugar when working on a break or wound. If the bird shows signs of increasing stress, such as heavy breathing, give the patient a few drops of the liquid and allow him a little time to settle down before continuing to work.

If an injured bird found in the wild needs restraining, cut a hole in a sock and place the bird within the sock with his head protruding through so that he may breathe. Then he should be placed in a covered box and kept warm until he may be brought to a place where treatment for his injuries can begin.

I always work from a sitting position with the bird on a bath towel in my lap. I have found this to be much easier than bending over a table. Just the slight pressure of the forearms holding the bird on the towel seems to quiet him. But beware of putting him further into shock.

The supplies needed to work on most injuries include: sterile gauze, half-inch adhesive tape, small scissors and tweezers, cardboard (shirt cardboard for small birds), disinfectant and ointment, towels and facial tissue. Place everything you need within easy reach on a table in front of you. Cut a few strips of tape and attach them to the table ready for instant use; (masking tape will remove fewer feathers). If you will need gauze pads with medication on them for use over open wounds, have them cut to proper size with medication already applied. Remember to keep a small glass of sweetened milk and a medicine dropper handy if the patient seems to be unusually disturbed.

A bird will need to be immobilized while you are applying a splint. With larger birds it is best to have someone else there to aid in holding. Tape the legs of predatory birds to be safe from razor-sharp talons. Holding birds during firstaid is an art in itself. With smaller birds it is awkward to have too many hands in the way, but it may nonetheless be necessary.

It is better to treat a bird without an audience. The bird will remain quiet if he cannot see your movements, so place a tissue lightly over the head to provide darkness without obstructing breathing. For a small bird use the foot of a nylon stocking with a hole cut for the wing or leg which is to be worked on, the head protruding through the toe of the stocking. Restrain the harmful gyrations of a larger bird by wrapping him in a piece of cloth cut large enough to cover his body with a hole through which to insert the injured wing or leg. Secure with safety pins firmly about the bird's body, taking care to leave the sheeting around the head loose enough for easy breathing. Sometimes with smaller birds a tissue merely placed over the head is sufficient to calm them and allow work on the injury. But be prepared to use the stocking to prevent further injury and the loss of that absolute calm which is necessary for successful healing.

I have heard it said that if you leave a bird with a broken leg alone, it will heal by itself. It probably will, and in many cases reasonably straight; however, this is taking an unnecessary chance. I have seen many birds with their legs healed in such an improper position that the legs were nearly useless. So if a bird is brought to you with a broken leg, apply a splint. For robins and quail this is doubly important, since they run on the ground for food. Various birds depend on different parts of their anatomy for specialized activities. Get to know your charge, read up on him immediately, seek expert advice as soon as possible.

Sometimes it is difficult to tell if a leg is broken. If the bird cannot flex his toes, there is a break, and with careful examination it can be found. Sometimes a bird will hit a car windshield or other hazard, bruising a leg so that he can't use it. This requires no splint, just rest and food until he is able to move properly. Often a bird will become entangled in a piece of string while building a nest, or fly into an abandoned kite string. As he hangs from the string and struggles to free himself, the joints may become sprained and bruised, and the leg will appear useless. Here again, no splint is necessary. I have seen string-entangled birds lacerate all the skin on their legs without breaking any bones. An application of antiseptic salve with gauze taped over the abrasion will soon heal it.

Don't be in a hurry to splint a bird's leg. Review what you are going to do and have everything in readiness before you start the splinting process. Firm, calm handling is essential, but don't overdo the firmness. Remember that the bones of airborne birds are hollow. As a result they are extremely fragile, and it is possible in handling a bird to break a bone accidentally. This fragility should also be taken into account when building cages for convalescents. Most ground birds' bones afford a bit more strength against breakage, and diving birds have yet more solid bones.

Food and water should always be kept on the floor of the cage for birds with broken wings or legs.

Broken Wings

A broken wing is a painful and dangerous injury for a bird to sustain. Repeated fluttering of the wing in an attempt to fly is injurious, and the inability to lift out of danger is frightening and creates a survival problem for the bird. A bird cannot use a wing that is out of joint or broken, or has a severe nerve injury. If broken, the wing will need a splint to heal properly. If the joint is out of place or a nerve injured, the wing will not need a splint but should be supported for comfort until it heals. A break will usually heal in two weeks in smaller birds, in large birds perhaps as much as six weeks. In the case of displacement, support may be required for only a few hours, or a day or two. A severe nerve injury could take longer than a break to heal. Here you will have to use your judgment by removing the support and letting the bird have freedom of movement to test his improvement.

When a bird's wing hangs loosely, lower than the other wing, it may very well be broken and will require splinting for proper healing. If the break is in the middle or near the tip of the wing, it can be done very easily. If the break is in a joint it might heal in a rigid position. You really have no way of telling what will happen, so it is best to proceed with the splinting and hope for the best.

I have found that splinting a simple wing break can be done in the same manner on all sizes of birds. The only variation is the use of wider pieces of tape and stiffer cardboard for larger birds. Don't weigh the bird down with matchsticks or other wood, except for balsa in the case of a break in a bird the size of a swan.

If there are no pieces of wing bone protruding from the skin, splint only one side of the wing, the underside. However, if the bone has broken through the skin, it is advisable to apply two splints, one to each side of the wing. When a bone is protruding, be sure to disinfect the wound thoroughly with alcohol, peroxide, or Phisohex. Carefully remove any feathers that might be in the wound with tweezers. Pull the skin together after setting the bone back in place, and cushion with gauze pads dabbed with ointment. Always apply the splint securely over such a break so that the bone is kept rigidly in place.

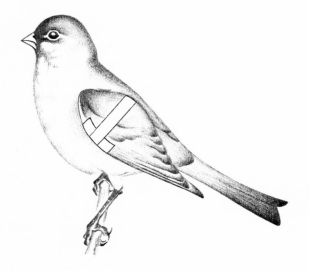

Simple Wing Break

Nature starts the healing process almost as soon as an injury occurs, so the sooner a break is splinted the better the chance of successful recovery. If a break is a few days old and bone is protruding, you may not be able to get the bone in place. In such a case it is best to have a veterinarian do the job. He will be able to use anesthesia to lessen the pain, as was the procedure with a huge barn owl once brought to me. The bones had started to heal and had crossed over from the pull of muscles and tendons. They had to be pulled apart and a pin inserted before splinting.

Always place gauze with medication directly next to a wound or break, and then apply the splint over the bandage. The splint may be wrapped with adhesive tape before application. This prevents the cardboard from disintegrating should it get wet. The bird will peck off a splint if the cardboard is softened by moisture.

It is advisable to measure the length of your splints against the uninjured wing so that you can cut them to the correct size and shape before applying. Cut adhesive tape to desired lengths, and hang it from the edge of the table for easy reach. Always cut more strips than you think you'll need so that if a piece loses adhesion you will have an immediate replacement.

Birds need their wings for balance as well as for flight, so unless the break is in the body joint, do not let the tape completely immobilize the wings. Quite often a bird will fall over on his side after a wing has been splinted. Do not be too concerned; soon he will become accustomed to the tape and will straighten up and learn to balance.

Breaks in a bird's wing usually occur at one or more of four places in the wing: between the wing tip and outer joint; in the outer joint; between the outer joint and the body joint; and in the body joint.

Wing Breaks—Between Wing Tip and Outer Joint; Outer Joint and Body Joint

If a break occurs between the wing tip and the outer joint, or the outer joint and the shoulder joint, tape a strip of cardboard over the break. Any open wounds will need to be cush-

ioned with gauze to which you have applied antiseptic ointment.

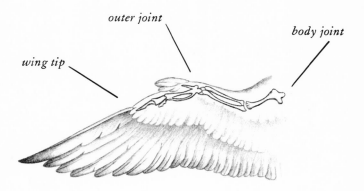

Wing Anatomy

Wing Breaks—Outer Joint

A contour splint is excellent if the break is in the outer
joint of the wing. It may also be used to reinforce the straight
type of splints which are applied if the break is between the
joints. You may have to cut several of these before you get
one that best fits the bird you are treating. Always use the
unbroken wing for measuring. Don't be discouraged: you'll be
all thumbs at first but it becomes easier with practice.

After the splint is folded on the dotted line, it can be inserted
under the wing, folded back over the wing and taped together,
both in front and in back of the joint. Tape should be crossed
the opposite way on the splint to secure the splint together over
the outer joint. Use cardboard from men's shirts for this splint:
it is lightweight and easily cut to fit.

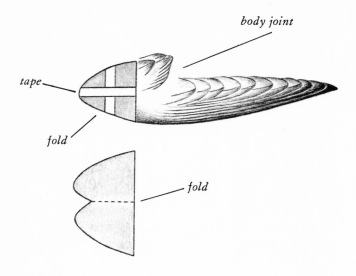

body joint

tape

fold

fold

Contour Splint

After you have cleaned, medicated and splinted the break, cut a piece of half-inch masking tape long enough to go completely around the bird's body with an inch extra for overlap. This will act as the anchor tape for supporting the break. Start on the bird's back between the wings and bring the tape under the wing, close to but not cutting into the joint. Bring it across the bird's chest and up under the other wing and lap the end of the tape over the starting point. Be sure the tape is pressed firmly around the bird's body, not tightly enough to hurt but so that it will not shift or turn. No matter where the break in the wing is, it will need to be supported by the body in this fashion.

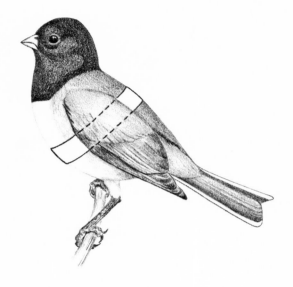

Anchor Tape

(For birds that are quite large you might want to use wider tape. However, I like the half-inch tape best since removing it pulls out fewer feathers than would a wider tape. When removing the tape, cut it into small sections.)

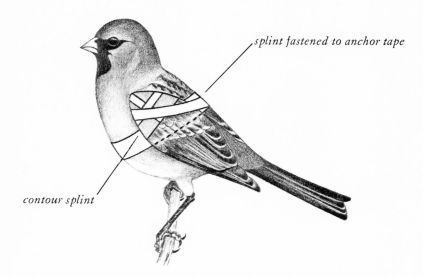

splint fastened to anchor tape

contour splint

Contour Splint Applied

After you have applied splints over the break and have bound the tape around the body, you are ready to anchor the broken wing to the body support. Cut a piece of tape long enough to go around the wing. Start in the middle of the back, over the tape you have already put around the body. Hold the tape, sticky side up, with the thumb and take the tape under the broken wing, folding the wing gently up against the body so that it seems to be in a natural position. Bring the tape back up over the wing and secure the end to the small sticky side at the starting point. Extend it down under the other wing so that it is fastened securely to the body support.

79

What results is simply a loop of tape around the naturally folded wing, fastened on top of the back to support the weight of the broken wing. The bird will still be able to lift his wing and balance himself.

If there is so much swelling that it is impossible to fold the wing into a natural position, fold it as well as possible without forcing it and then give support. The support can be tightened as the swelling decreases.

Wing Breaks—Body Joint

If the break is in the body joint it cannot be splinted. However, it must be rigidly supported. This is the most painful break since the whole weight of the wing will pull against the break. Often the area of the bird's body around such a break will be swollen and discolored from internal bleeding. The first step is to place the anchor tape around the bird's body. Next, using antiseptic ointment on a piece of gauze, fit it gently under the bird's wing so that it covers the irritated area. Follow the same support procedure as if it had a contour splint on the injured wing and anchor it to the supporting tape around the body. Because the break is at the body joint, you will want to immobilize the wing further by fastening another piece of tape on the supporting tape under the body, bringing it back up over the injured wing, and fastening it to the anchor tape on top of the body.

After about two weeks, cut this last piece of tape in one place only, at the bottom of the wing. This will allow the bird to begin exercising the wing joint without putting any real pressure on it. Leave the loop around the wing and the supporting tape on the bird for at least another week before removing.

Recuperation After Wing Breaks and Nerve Injuries

As soon as initial mending is over—ten days to two weeks, longer for body joint breaks—the bird should be given quarters large enough for freedom of movement. Perches should be placed at opposite ends of the quarters and at varying heights so that he can start exercising the wing.

Broken wings are not always as successfully mended as broken legs. If the break is in a joint it may heal rigidly. If it is properly supported and does heal stiffly it will at least be in a natural position and not hinder movement. The bird may not be able to fly, or he may fly poorly, but he will be able to balance with the wing and it will afford him some help in getting around. With time and practice he may learn to navigate well enough to take very good care of himself. A robin whose whole wing had been amputated spent several happy years in the enclosed yard of one of my kind-hearted friends. The bird was given sour cherries, ground beef, bread and blueberries for winter fare, when the worm and bug population waned; but otherwise he foraged for himself, chased other robins around the yard during mating season, bathed in his low water dish and generally ruled the yard.

Foot Splints

Measure the bird's foot from the end of the back toe to the tip of the longest front toe. Cut the splint from cardboard to form a pie-shaped wedge. Then cut out the V-shaped areas between the toes, and cut smaller V-shaped areas for the toenails to fit into.

Depending on the size of the bird, split adhesive tape into narrow strips long enough to apply over the foot and fasten to the splint. Crisscross the strips of tape so that the toes are held separately in their respective slots. This gives a more

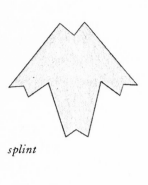

splint

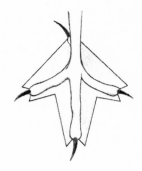

foot on splint (top view)

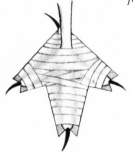

continuous tape around splint

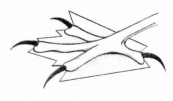

foot on splint (side view)

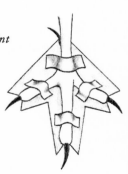

splint taped in place

Foot Splints

82

natural position to the bird's foot and will be more comfortable. Never pry the bird's toes too far apart; approximate the natural position of the foot. You can determine this configuration by placing the bird's uninjured foot firmly on a piece of cardboard and outlining the toes with a pencil. Be sure the toenails are left uncovered in each slot. This is a sure way to see that each toe is properly in place.

I sometimes place several thicknesses of gauze between the bottom of the bird's foot and the splint to act as a cushion.

Be sure the pieces of tape are applied in such a way that the entire splint is covered by a continuous piece of tape. This prevents moisture from ruining the splint. It may be necessary to run a strip of adhesive from the splint around the bird's ankle. Do not use more gauze and adhesive than is absolutely necessary, as the splint needs to be kept lightweight.

Keep a firm hold on the leg while carefully removing the splint to avoid cutting the foot.

Broken Legs

Preparation of any wound before applying splints or dressings is the same: clean the wound to disinfect it, and use sterile gauze dressed with antiseptic salve. Feathers on the edges of wounds should be removed. Have a glass of disinfectant with a medicine dropper in it for easy application to the wound. A wound can be disinfected again later without disturbing the splint and gauze by carefully inserting a medicine dropper and squeezing the disinfectant over the wound.

Always cut splints from cardboard. I have found after trying many substitutes that this is the best material. Use balsa wood, which is light and easy to shape, as a reinforcement to the cardboard splint only when treating large birds such as swans, ducks, geese, large hawks and owls.

Complete immobilization is vital while applying a leg

splint. There are several ways to do this, depending on the size and type of bird. Since it is very hard to work on a bird of the smaller species with someone else holding, run a piece of narrow tape around the wings and body to fetter him. A small bath towel laid between the legs will hold the good leg down while giving support to the broken leg. The most convenient way is to lay the bird on its side on a bath towel in your lap. Have all the equipment needed on a table in front of you.

Cut the pieces of tape you will need and hang them down from the table's edge for handy use. It may be necessary to shield the bird's face with a piece of tissue to lessen the fright.

Sometimes it is difficult to discover just where a break is on the leg. It could be a cracked bone, or possibly only a nerve injury or bad bruise. In any case, if the leg hangs limp and useless it is best to apply the splint and not take the chance of further injury.

As previously mentioned, if the bird seems especially frightened, stop working on the injury and give him a few drops of milk from an eyedropper. Let him rest a few moments before proceeding.

Be extremely careful when working with taloned birds such as hawks and owls. Secure the leg that is not broken so the bird will not be able to strike with it. Those talons can penetrate to the bone, so have another person wearing gloves help in holding.

When measuring a bird's leg for the size of splint needed, use the good leg. Measure the distance from the bird's ankle to just behind the elbow, then from below the elbow to the top of the body joint. For a bird the size of a sparrow make the splint one inch longer than measurement from below the elbow to the top of the body joint. In larger birds it will need to be proportionately longer to allow the splint to come well up over the joint for a more rigid position.

If the injury is in the ankle area, cut the splint with a sharper upward angle to hold the bird's foot well up from the ground. If the foot is held up in this manner the ankle will usually heal without any other support.

For large birds, where wood is needed for reinforcement, the cardboard splint must be cut to proper size first, and completely covered with tape; then also cover the wood completely with tape. Tape the wood to the outside of the splint. A pair of scissors may be used to cut a tongue depressor or balsa wood to the right length. For larger birds the adhesive tape should be one inch in width; use the half-inch width for smaller birds. In splinting very small birds like hummingbirds, chickadees, and kinglets I have found it necessary to split the tape to less than the half-inch width.

The usual leg break needs only a few weeks to heal. However, where there are bones protruding through the skin, it may take longer. In such cases it is sometimes best to remove the splint in sections, leaving the part that is directly over the wound until last. When a break has healed the bird will be able to flex its toes. Although you may notice the toes moving slightly after just a few days, leave the splint on for a full two weeks; this allows the bone to heal more solidly. Be very careful not to let a splinted bird get away from you. The tape will remain to endanger the bird for many weeks.

Leg Breaks—Elbow Splints

No matter where the break is in the leg, use the elbow type of splint shown. This splint enables the bird to perch, sit flat on the ground or move about without the broken leg getting in the way. The bird will soon learn to balance on the elbow of the splint when either perching or on the ground. The cardboard is lightweight so he can fly with the leg splinted. It is the only kind of splint that will completely immobilize the broken leg and permit an uninterrupted healing process.

Before applying the splint, treat any open wounds on the leg with disinfectant and apply a piece of gauze with healing ointment. Wrap the leg entirely in gauze to keep the tape from adhering to the leg.

Cut the splint at an angle to let the bird balance on the elbow without causing the foot to rest on the ground. This keeps the foot free of abrasion and prevents disturbance to the break. Splints should always be placed on the outer side of the leg and reinforced with adhesive tape running the full length of the splint. If a bone is protruding through the skin, strengthen the mend with a narrow length of cardboard on the underneath side of the leg.

Leave room for some swelling when binding up the splint, and examine the leg each day. If swelling has occurred and the bandage seems too tight, simply cut through the tape to release the tension, and reattach the now-separated ends with a small piece of tape. Be sure the splint does not rub or protrude against the bird's foot, causing irritation or swelling in the ankle area.

If there is an open wound, do not place so much tape around the leg at the point of injury that you are unable to reach the wound: with a small medicine dropper apply liquid disinfectant each day until you are sure there is no infection. Thoroughly wet the gauze around the wound with medication.

When the break is between the body joint and the elbow of the leg, start a piece of tape at the elbow, bring it up the splint and under the wings, over the back, down across the chest, and fasten it to the splint.

If the break is between the foot and elbow, cut the splint with a tab extending from the lower end. Roll the tab over a pencil or round stick. The broken leg will fit into the rolled tab. When the tape is applied around the leg the break will be supported on all sides. The tab is not needed if the break is in the upper leg.

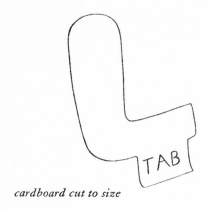

cardboard cut to size

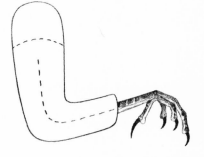

splint rolled to fit leg

Elbow Splint

For a break between foot and elbow the lower portion of the elbow splint is cut with a tab extending downward, as you will note in the illustrations. When a piece of adhesive tape the exact width of the tab is taped to it, the tab may be brought under the lower portion of the leg and then fastened back up over the splint. This forms a cradle for the leg to rest in. After the tape has been fastened to the tab, use a pencil to roll the tab around so that it will conform to the shape of the bird's leg.

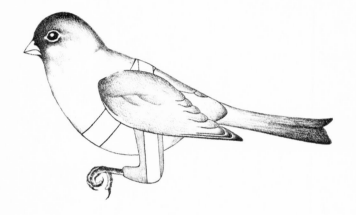

Elbow Splint Applied

Note that the tape is placed along the length of the splint and around the bird's body to support a break in the upper leg. The bird can perch with the injured leg held up out of the way. He can also lower himself with the elbow of the splint resting on the perch for balance.

Leg Breaks—Circle Splints

The circle splint is applied only to reinforce an elbow splint, mainly in cases where broken segments overlap or have slipped to the sides. When this occurs it may be difficult to hold the bones together while taping up the elbow splint, and a circle splint should be put on the break before the elbow splint is applied.

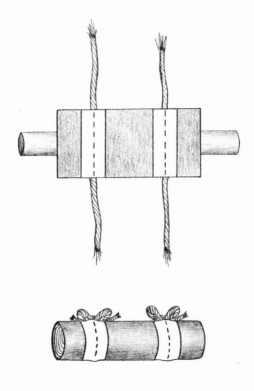

Circle Splints

The circle splint is much like a corset—it can be brought together by pulling the strings and tying them, or loosened by untying them. The circumference of the circle splint is determined by measuring the good leg. It needs to be small enough so that when the strings are drawn together the edges of the cardboard do not quite meet, and long enough to extend well above and below the break. Tape two pieces of small, stout string to the cardboard. Roll the splint on a round object so it will readily fit the contour of the leg. Tie the ends of string in a bow knot. The splint must not be drawn too tightly; this will be painful to the bird and swelling will surely occur around the break.

After the splint has been applied, gently turn it so the knot is facing the back of the leg if the break is in the upper leg. If the break is in the lower leg, turn the splint so the strings are tied toward the front of the leg. These positions allow you to adjust the knot easily in case of swelling. By clipping the tape which holds the elbow splint, the strings may be untied and loosened without removing the splint or disturbing the break.

If there is a break in the skin on the upper leg, it bears repeating that medication must be applied before any splint. Always wrap gauze around the lower leg to prevent the tape from sticking to the leg.

The splints should conform to the positions indicated. Remember to apply the elbow splint *over* the circle splint and to examine splints each day for swelling.

Both Legs Broken

About eight birds with both legs broken have been brought to me for repair during my years of working with birds. While they require more care during convalescence, the birds adapt very readily to being immobilized, heal just as rapidly, and in most ways react to the double injury as though it were one. However, if one break is more severe than the other it may be necessary to leave that splint on longer.

The method of splinting is the same as for one break. After the legs are splinted a simple cardboard support is applied.

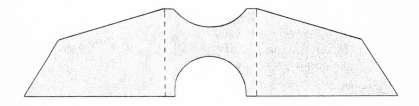

Cardboard Support
(cardboard should be heavier
than that used for splint)

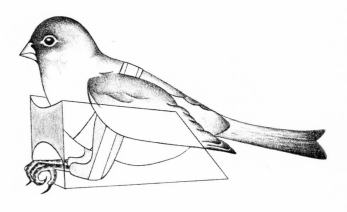

Both Legs Splinted & Supported

The bird should be kept in a large box, not in a cage. Tissue should be packed lightly around him to prevent tipping over, and food and water put in front for easy reach. A large bird may need heavier toweling for stabilization. Use tissues under and around the bird for cleanliness and easy disposal. A screen may be placed over the box so that the bird will not attempt to fly about.

SPRAWLED LEGS

Sometimes young birds' legs will protrude to the sides of their bodies rather than maintain a straight and natural position beneath them. This may be caused by their position in the nest but more likely it is a result of dietary deficiency, nerve damage, or a hereditary tendency. I have found that by supporting the legs with tape this condition can sometimes be helped. Simply run narrow adhesive tape over the legs near the top joint and around the body; this will give just enough support to keep the legs in a natural and comfortable position while the bird is gaining strength. Supplement the diet with vitamins. In severe cases it may be necessary to place an additional strip of adhesive under the body and around each leg. Check daily that the tape is not too tight or too loose, but just firm enough for support. If the sprawled condition is caused by severe deformity, temporary taping probably will not help. However it may alleviate the condition enough so that the bird will be able to get around.

The first figure shows tape across chest, over both legs and fastened on top of bird's back. If only one leg is sprawled, tape can be used in same way but going under the uninjured leg. In second figure, tape may be used in same way, around both legs holding them together in natural position, or around just one leg and then around the body keeping the one leg in place. Two weeks should remedy the fault. First tape is below

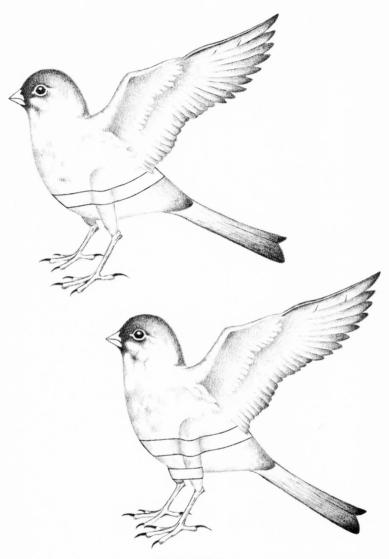

Sprawled Legs

the top leg joint; second tape is just above second joint and kept close under and against the bird's stomach.

BROKEN BEAKS

A broken beak poses a problem of survival for any bird. Unless his beak is repaired and supported and he is hand-fed until the injury heals, the bird will die of starvation. Most breaks heal within ten days to two weeks, so the hand-feeding process takes less time than that required to raise a young bird.

In some instances a support on the beak will enable the bird to feed himself. This depends on where the break is and whether or not the bird has enough control to open and shut his beak. Breaks seldom occur in the upper beak. This half of the mouth is part of the bird's skull and does not move, whereas the lower, movable part of the beak is much more vulnerable to injury. One exception is the skimmer, whose upper beak is hinged.

After any injury the beak will be quite sore for a few days and the bird will be very reluctant to use it. Hand-feeding may be necessary for a short time, until the soreness subsides and the bird regains use of his beak. Feed at least every few hours or he will become weak.

If the bird can feed himself, soft food should be placed in a container wide enough for feeding without the beak hitting the sides. The container should be twice as deep as the length of the bird's beak so that he will be able to dip into the food without touching the broken beak to the hard surface. Water should be put in a similar vessel and both containers kept well filled.

The beak may only be cracked and if so will not need support. If damage of this type occurs at the side where the beak is attached to the head, the beak will benefit from a couple of stitches to hold it in place.

Allowing the beak to heal out of alignment will limit the bird's ability to pick up food. Be sure the repair job brings the upper and lower beaks firmly together and in line with each other.

It is almost impossible to repair a broken beak with adhesive tape, which becomes moist during feeding and drinking and loses its adhesion. The only practical method of repair is to sew a waterproof support to the beak. This is a very difficult procedure. A lightweight rustproof and waterproof support must be firmly attached to the break. The wound is left open so that it may be easily cleaned and disinfected. The support is sewn into the tissue of the beak itself, an extremely delicate procedure: the support must be fastened with thread wrapped several times around the beak and must not interfere with the action of the bird's tongue. I advise that a veterinarian perform this operation to minimize the stress and possible additional injuries. The counsel of veterinarians and members of your local Humane Society should always be sought when treating intricate disorders like this.

MUSCULAR WEAKNESS IN THE NECK

Sometimes birds have trouble with the muscles holding the neck upright. You may be able to correct this by applying a small cardboard splint from the side of the neck to the top of the head. Tape it in place with very narrow pieces of adhesive, taking care not to choke the bird. Do not cross the nostrils and cut off breathing, and be cautious when working close to the eyes.

BB SHOT AND PELLET WOUNDS

BB shot, or airgun or shotgun pellets often force feathers into the wound, and hardened blood holds the shot inside. Examine injured birds thoroughly for dislocated feathers or knots on the body which may indicate such a wound. Soften the area with warm water or salve, then gently remove the feathers with tweezers. If you cannot readily see the shot, direct a flashlight beam into the wound. Sometimes the pellet can be located this way, but you may have to probe for it. Cleanse and thoroughly disinfect the wound, and leave it open for drainage but protected from flies.

AIR BUBBLES

If a bird flies into something or is dealt a blow, an air bubble may form as a result of an internal body rupture which allows air to gather under the skin. Sometimes the bubble will form near the leg or under a wing and cause the leg to extend to the side or the wing to extend at an exaggerated angle. If the bubble forms around the neck area the bird's head may be forced to one side. It is uncomfortable to the bird wherever it occurs and the pressure should be relieved. This is easily accomplished by the use of a needle that has been sterilized. Insert the tip of the needle under the skin where the bubble has formed and exert just enough upward pressure to hold the hole open to release the air. Be careful to insert the needle just barely under the skin and be very gentle with the upward pressure. Keep the bird quiet for an hour or so, then re-examine to be sure that no other bubbles have been formed. If they have, repeat the process. Put a little antiseptic ointment over the area you have punctured. When you are sure no more bubbles will form, release the bird.

SUTURES

A wound which commonly requires suturing will be on the crop (the neck pouch of doves and some other birds). Elsewhere on the body it may be possible to disinfect the wound, draw it together and bandage it with gauze and tape so that it heals. But the crop will spill out food and water if there is an opening, and the bird will become dehydrated and starve.

Sewing up a wound is very simple. You may feel squeamish

when attempting the suture, thinking each stitch must give the bird pain, but this need not be so. If you work carefully and calmly, your patient will hardly feel the process. It is best to have a veterinarian do the job, but the average person can make a satisfactory repair if he prepares for the suture first and uses common sense.

The most convenient way to work on a patient is to sit in a chair with a towel on your lap. Lay the bird or animal on the towel. All medicine and equipment should be directly in front of you on a table within easy reach. Cut any adhesive you might need and secure the strips to the edge of the table. You will need a suture needle (a small, curved upholstery needle can be substituted), silk thread or even dental floss, scissors, half-inch wide adhesive tape, tweezers, a small glass of disinfectant (alcohol, Phisohex, or peroxide), a medicine dropper, gauze, and antiseptic salve.

The bird must be immobile while you are suturing. You will need both hands for the job and anyone trying to hold the bird may be in the way. Wrap the body firmly in a towel or some other material long enough to go around the patient several times. Leave the area to be sutured free, and be sure the bird can breathe freely while covered lightly by a tissue to calm him.

Have the disinfectant ready, thread the needle, and then drop it into the cup of disinfectant until ready to use.

Use tweezers to remove any feathers inside or along the edge of the wound. Using scissors gently snip off any ragged pieces of flesh around the wound, then clean it with disinfectant that has been somewhat diluted.

Only the edges of the wound need to be caught with the needle. With the index finger and thumb of one hand gently press the edges of the wound together while you draw the thread through with the other hand. This should keep the thread from tearing holes in the edges of the wound. Stitches should be only about one-sixth of an inch apart. Leave about three inches of free thread at each end of the wound; these may be tied together later to keep the threads from coming loose.

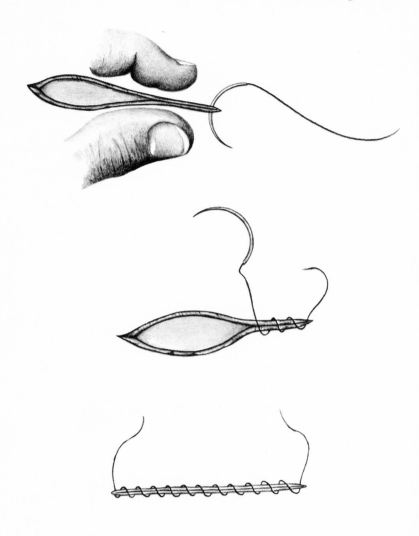

Suturing

Sewing Directions: If you are right-handed, sew from right to left so that the forefinger and thumb of the left hand may be used to draw the wound gently together as the thread is being tightened with each stitch. This prevents the thread from tearing through the flesh as the stitches are drawn together. Always use the basic whipping stitch. Don't knot the end of the thread, but be sure to leave several inches of thread free at each end of the wound so they may be tied together after the stitching is completed.

After you have completed the suture, drop antiseptic from the medicine dropper over the area. Fold gauze large enough to cover the wound several times and put antiseptic ointment on it. Illustration shows how to bind the gauze over the sutured area with two long strips of tape, continuing the tape around the bird's body so the gauze will remain firmly in place.

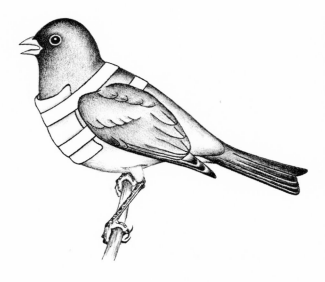

Bandaged Wound

Leave the stitches in for ten days to two weeks, depending on the nature of the wound. Then clip the stitches, remove them with tweezers, and disinfect the wound again. Wait a few days before releasing to be sure the wound is completely healed.

OLD WOUNDS

If a wound is a day or so old, the attendant blood and feathers may have become so matted and dried that it is impossible to suture immediately. In this case, draw the wound together as best you can and tape gauze, with a generous amount of antiseptic salve on it, tightly over the wound. Leave this on for a few hours until the salve has had a chance to soften the feathers somewhat. Then remove the gauze and clean the wound before suturing.

A bird who has sustained a crop wound is usually dehydrated from constant loss of liquids, so give water immediately. If the bird is weak it is best to give the milk and sugar mixture. Even if the wound has only been taped and not yet sutured the bird will be able to retain some of the liquid. After the bird has regained some of his strength, place food and water in front of him and see if he tries to eat. Do not force-feed solid food to a bird with a ruptured crop; if he eats voluntarily it is all right.

AMPUTATIONS

Never be in a hurry to amputate. Although you may feel absolutely sure that the nerves and blood vessels have been severed and that the limb will be lost, it is best to wait. Do a repair job; a crippled limb may result but it will afford more balance than no limb at all. Examine the wound daily: a dying limb will become stiff and dry, there will probably be an odor, and the limb will have to be removed. Consult an expert before any amputation.

To amputate, first tie off the limb with a piece of strong thread, dental floss or string just above the live area to prevent bleeding. Cut away the limb below the tie-off. Thoroughly disinfect the stub, apply healing ointment on a cushion of gauze, and tape it firmly in place over the stub. It is important not to remove the tie-off string—it will come off later with the dressing.

Leave the gauze on for two weeks to give the wound a chance to heal over with a cushion of tissue. Remove the dressing; if the area still appears to be tender, apply a new dressing containing disinfectant powder instead of ointment.

Sometimes it is necessary to amputate a bird's wing because it is too badly mangled to recover. I had to do this with an owl who had tangled with a barbed wire fence. The owl was completely torn up, especially the wing. As it turned out I had to put him to sleep because a bit of the barbed wire had gone into his eye and he had lost the use of his foot.

MERCY KILLING

For those birds and small animals so hopelessly ill or injured that they are beyond help, the most humane act is to put them to sleep, ending their suffering. But the need to do so should be left up to an expert.

Ether or chloroform should be used, as the procedure is less painful than the use of a large needle containing a killing drug. Do it as soon as possible. If you do not have chloroform or ether, a veterinarian can phone a prescription to the nearest pharmacist for the amount needed.

Use an airtight receptacle large enough to hold the animal or bird without crowding it. A paper bag, tight cardboard container, or a cooking pan with an airtight cover will do. Put crumpled tissue on the bottom of the receptacle, place the patient on the tissue, pour the chloroform or ether on a tissue or piece of cloth, place it beside the creature, and then tightly close the receptacle and leave it alone for ten minutes. The darkness has a calming effect on the animal and the procedure is painless.

Do *not* use chloroform as an anesthetic for treating a wounded bird or animal.

Chapter 6

TREATMENT FOR POISONING
AND SHOCK

PESTICIDES

The production and marketing of pesticides is big business, and unfortunately the dollar sign tends to obscure more important signs in the environment. The gardener is sold a vision of beautiful lawns and a wealth of blossoms made easy with chemicals, but it's seldom pointed out that the insects and worms he poisons are eaten by birds. Seeds poisoned by weed killers are eaten by both birds and small mammals, and poisoned vegetation may be consumed by rabbits and other small herbivores. Even domestic animals do not escape this poison. Cats or dogs may walk across a lawn so treated, lick their paws, and become ill.

Every householder and gardener could help put a stop to this wholesale killing of wildlife by refusing to use preparations which are toxic to animals and birds. The federal government should remove these pesticides from the market. After all, the best insecticide comes in a feathered container.

At this writing I know of no sure cure for a bird that has been poisoned by pesticides. If the bird can be captured immediately after eating the poison, a long period of continuous dosing with vegetable oil and milk helps absorb some of the poison and eliminate it from the bird's system. However, by the time a bird is sick enough to be captured the poison is often all through the system and is very difficult to counteract. Activated charcoal mixed with milk and oil, given three or four times an hour, may pull him through. I have saved a number of birds with Uni-dote, a charcoal-based preparation sold in some drugstores. Milk of magnesia too may be of aid.

In 1961, many birds poisoned by pesticides were brought to me. The birds were of all varieties, but I kept records of only the robins, thirty of which died within a two-month period. Since the birds were found in widely scattered areas I assume that the poisons came from the average toxified home garden. I believe it takes only eleven poisoned earthworms to kill a robin. Robins feed these worms to their babies, endangering their lives, too; or, if the parents die of poisoning, the nestlings starve to death.

The symptoms are nearly the same in all poisoned birds. The bird becomes weak, refuses to eat, and loses the use of its legs as the attack on the nervous system intensifies. Sometimes convulsions precede death. If you are absolutely sure it is progressive poisoning, where repeated dosing of oil, milk, and activated charcoal yields no response, the kindest thing is to put the bird painlessly to sleep.

Spraying fruit trees like the mulberry for bagworms will cause the death of robins, mockingbirds, jays or any of the birds which eat fruit.

POISONS

Do not use rat poison, since it can be carried by the rat, dropped in the feces, and eaten by other animals.

Until research has developed sprays for garden use that are not toxic to bird or animal, the gardener could help to lessen the danger from poisons by rejecting the use of pesticides. I specifically refer to the application of insect sprays and crabgrass killers which kill thousands of birds each year. Read the "small print" on labels to see whether ingestion is fatal to an-

imals and birds. The manufacturers and sellers of these sprays
and powders have demonstrated little concern with their mis-
use and residual effects.

Attracting birds with feeders, bird houses, and landscaping
is the best way to control the bug population. At Point Reyes
Bird Observatory, California, the nest of a Wilson's warbler
was recently observed from dawn to dusk. The parents made
over 800 trips to the nest, carrying on the average five insects.
That's four thousand insects per day just for the nestlings; what
the parents ate was not observed. If the young are fed at this
rate for ten to fourteen days, one brood will consume about fifty
thousand insects!

SHOCK

Shock, "a rude unhinging of the machinery of life," is one
of the most common conditions in injured birds. In this state
the bird may be limp and unconscious. Stress from fear will
put a bird into shock. A bird that has been mauled by a cat will
die as often from shock as from the injury. Shock is often due
to a blow on the head or a fall, but if not otherwise injured too
badly the bird will most likely recover. Often birds fly into windows and are temporarily stunned. A drawn window shade will
usually alter the window's reflection so that birds will avoid it.
If a window is in the back of the house, where you would not
mind the appearance of a piece of screen or chicken wire, this
will effectively curb a bird's flight into the window. If it is on
ground floor level, a rose trellis may be leaned against the window as an indication to the bird that there is a barrier.

The first thing to do for shock cases is to line a small box with
tissues. Do not use cotton or the bird may get his feet entangled;
also, the box will be more difficult to clean. Check the bird for
other injuries, like leg or wing breaks or open abrasions, and
then test whether or not he can swallow by dripping a little milk

down his throat with a medicine dropper. If he does not swallow, do not force-feed him or he will choke. If he can swallow, feed him small amounts at frequent intervals. Check the food charts for the proper food.

Keep birds in shock in a secluded, warm, dry place. As they recover consciousness, they usually flop and stagger about. If they fly at all, it is very unsteadily. Cover open boxes with screen to prevent flight and further injury. Sometimes their sight is affected also, but unless there is eye damage proper vision will return, and as their equilibrium improves they will fly properly. When a patient flies with ease in the outside flight cage and can fend for himself in his natural surroundings, release him as near as possible to the place where he was found.

Confining a bird or animal in an area where he is constantly exposed to a source of light or heat which he cannot elude may also create the stress that induces shock. Don't leave an exposed light bulb in a cage or give too much heat. Allow the choice to move toward or away from heat or light. Handling or loud noises may also induce shock. Take care of your patients in an atmosphere of calm. Give them warmth, quiet, food and water. Stress impairs a creature's ability to heal himself, and when all is said and done it is mostly the patient who is the healer.

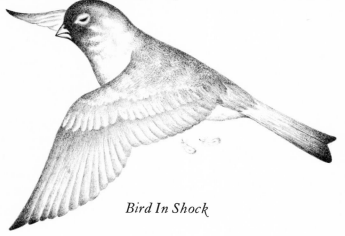

Bird In Shock

Chapter 7

TREATMENT FOR DISEASES

PNEUMONIA

Many injured birds die of pneumonia rather than from wounds they have sustained. Baby birds are especially vulnerable. The need of fledglings for warmth and protection from drafts or constant heat is paramount.

The same holds true for mature injured birds. Never place a wild bird or animal in an air-conditioned room or subject a bird to drastic changes of temperature. A bird that has been recuperating in a temperate room should not abruptly be moved outside on the first sunny day. It may seem warm to you, but a chill underlying the brightness of the sunshine could weaken the patient.

The first symptom of pneumonia is sudden loss of appetite and listlessness. When this occurs, keep the bird warm and give it a drop of whiskey in a jigger of water. This is not a cure but a stopgap measure until you are able to procure the proper medicine from a local pet store or veterinarian. An excellent medicine to keep on hand is Avimycin. Another indispensable medicine in the treatment of respiratory diseases is Hetacin-K. It is effective for congestion, tonsillitis, enteritis and bronchial pneumonia. To make breathing easier use a vaporizer with a medicine recommended by your vet. I usually add Vicks salve to the water in the vaporizer, making sure not to place it too near the patient.

HEPATITIS

In the fall, a lot of sparrows and other small birds develop a sort of hepatitis. They can't fly and are very weak, but they can pick up food from the ground. They are on their last legs, actually dying, and there isn't anything you can do for them. I've picked up many and taken care of them until they died, usually the next day. The larger birds apparently hide and you don't find them until they are dead, but smaller birds often stay about and are found incapacitated on a lawn.

BOTULISM

Botulism or "limber neck" is a kind of food poisoning that sometimes decimates whole populations of water birds, particularly ducks and geese. The seriousness of avian botulism increases as man continues to develop a million acres a year in the U.S. Increased concentration of wildlife populations in available habitat—as in the case of ducks, higher intensities of population in sloughs and marshes not yet drained or toxified by man—creates the situation where a disease or endemic killer such as botulism can kill fifty thousand ducks, as happened in a California slough in 1971. You may remember that photo of a mountain of dead ducks about to be cremated.

Botulism is caused by a toxin released from a bacterium that thrives in the gut of invertebrates, particularly maggots. Recent research indicates that birds acquire botulism by eating maggots living in the lethal toxins of other dead birds, and that it is not found, as originally presumed, in living vegetation or organically rich mud. When a bird is found suffering from botulism it is usually in critical condition. Paralysis prevents the nerves from transmitting messages to the muscle tissues. Flush out the intestinal tract with an Epsom salt solution administered orally. If it is a large bird such as a duck, a small basting syringe may be used. Otherwise fifteen-minute intervals of dosing with milk of magnesia from an eyedropper will be necessary. When using Epsom salts a bird must be given water to replace the dehydration which occurs within twenty minutes. Birds flushed out every six hours with this solution seem to improve. Antitoxins have been developed and should soon become available. Between treatments their natural diet should be offered. Those unable to eat should be given liquid nourishment. Normal husbandry methods should be followed, shade provided and the birds wet down periodically. Birds who regain their muscular control may be released once they have demonstrated a couple days' normal behavior.

DUTCH DUCK PLAGUE

Dutch duck plague was first reported in the western hemisphere in 1967 and was thought to be contained, since no outbreak of this disease was recorded west of Pennsylvania. But in April 1972 ducks and geese swimming in the lagoon of San Francisco's Palace of Fine Arts began dying. Considerable laboratory research showed that the diseased birds were infected with duck virus enteritis commonly known as Dutch duck plague. Apparently the extensive efforts on the east coast to prevent the spread of this disease had failed. Perhaps the disease has infected populations of migratory birds.

At this writing no cure has yet been developed. To determine if the disease has spread to other members of a population requires a complex quarantine system: pens must be cleaned, floors mopped, extensive records kept, and a control of other non-infected birds maintained. As with any birds found dying in appreciable numbers, a victim should be taken to the local Humane Society where it may be forwarded to a wildlife laboratory for examination to find the cause. If you suspect a bird is suffering from a communicable disease, you should quarantine it from the other patients you are treating.

ASPERGILLOSIS

One of the major killers of captive water birds is aspergillosis, a common mold or fungus found in decaying vegetable matter. For this reason straw is not recommended as a litter for the pens of rehabilitating water birds. Infections of this fungus in humans are rare, but it is deadly to wildlife populations. Investigations suggest that spores of this fungus, found in nearly all healthy birds, become dangerous when a bird's resistance is lowered or the incidence of airborne fungus spores becomes exceedingly high. Typically, inhaled spores succeed in germinating on the bird's air sac and in its lung tissue. As the fungus grows into a fuzzy mass it blocks the bird's respiratory passages. The bird's breathing creates a danger of infection to other birds by the airborne spores. Death often results from a combination of factors including impaired functioning of the lungs, loss of elasticity of the air sacs, and the effects of the toxin.

A bird may be rendered susceptible to aspergillosis by almost any kind of stress: nutritional, thermal, psychological, hormonal, or chemical. Insufficient salt intake or a molt may weaken some captive birds, which are already stressed due to their captivity, to the point where they contract aspergillosis. Certainly the best way to prevent a healthy bird from being afflicted by this disease is to leave it in the wild. If, however, it is necessary to keep a bird in captivity (especially a seabird) take care that the bird not be exposed to any material such as straw or hay which might be a medium for this mold. Pens sprayed with a one percent copper sulfate solution seem less susceptible to its growth. It is important to minimize and counteract stress so this disease does not overtake water birds kept in captivity resultant from such emergencies as an oil spill or botulism.

If an infected bird shows the symptoms of difficulty of breathing, weight loss, coughing or a sneezing or rattling sound in breathing, immediately quarantine him from the other birds and go to a veterinarian for the most recently developed medications. There is controversy about the means to cure this fungal affliction, as yet no single substance seems to have come forth.

TRICHOMONIASIS

My first experience with trichomoniasis, which is found in doves, pigeons, turkeys and sometimes in other species of birds, was with a young brown thrasher I had raised and released who came back at the end of summer to die of this disease.

Detailed information is available through the United States Fish and Wildlife Service in Washington, D.C., but I will give you a brief description of the disease so that you will recognize it if you discover a bird so infected.

Trichomoniasis is a fungus-like growth, yellow in color, always accompanied by a bad odor from the bird's mouth. If it is not discovered and treated at an early stage, it will develop to such an extent that the bird can no longer swallow and will starve to death. Even though badly infected, the bird may still have the strength to fly away when approached. Birds in this deteriorating condition should be put to sleep to relieve their suffering and to eliminate further spread of the disease, which is contagious. Trichomoniasis may start its growth at any point from the crop to the beak of the bird. I have seen birds with their tongues eaten away, crops filled with the disease, or a hard knot the size of a marble in the middle of the neck. A bird with any of these readily noticeable symptoms might well be put to sleep.

The disease may spread through drinking water or, in the case of doves and pigeons, through their method of feeding the young. It is not communicable to humans.

Trichomoniasis can be treated with a medicine called Enheptin. Consult a veterinarian, who will know the proper dosage and how to administer it. The newer medicines are Emtryl,

Hepcide, and Ipropran which I understand is quite effective. Enheptin is still used but the newer medicines may be easier to obtain. Of fifteen collared doves in an aviary, only the one in an advanced stage of the disease died. Of the remaining doves, ten showed the disease cultures taken from their throats. Treated with Enheptin, none of these died.

I think I might have infected this group of doves by releasing an infected, injured wild dove into their midst for convalescence. After the wild dove recovered I released it, not knowing that it carried the disease. Later I learned always to examine the crop, throat and mouth of a dove or pigeon for abnormal thickness which might indicate the growth, or the offensive odor which accompanies trichomoniasis.

RABIES

I am always amazed when adults encourage a child to touch, feed or attempt to pick up a wild animal. The automatic response of a wild animal is to protect itself by biting or scratching. Then the child's parent becomes frightened of rabies. Any warm-blooded animal can have this disease, so infection is a possibility whether the bite comes from a bat, mouse, raccoon, chipmunk, squirrel or any animal. Never let a child hand a peanut to a squirrel. Even though the little animal means well, it may accidentally nip the hand that feeds it. Drop the food and let the animal pick it up.

In many instances a wild animal may have some disease other than rabies; it may be so sick that it should be put to sleep immediately to end its suffering. However, if it has bitten someone it must be quarantined for at least ten days or until it dies, so that it can be examined for rabies. Frequently the place of quarantine is unhealthy, the food is improper, and medication is often not supplied. The animal may have convulsions from an illness other than rabies, and too often no sedatives are administered to relieve this suffering. If quarantine is required for a female animal with dependent babies, during the ten-day period her babies could starve to death.

One should always remember that wild animals are afraid of humans. If an animal appears tame its normality can be questioned and rabies suspected. Should a person be bitten it is important to capture the animal and immediately see a doctor.

Sometimes an animal crossing a highway may be hit by a car and stunned. If a thoughtful person cares enough to give assistance to the animal he should not try to touch or lift the animal without bite-proof gloves, perhaps a blanket wrapped around the animal, or some other means of lifting the animal without chancing a bite. The animal in its dazed condition may appear to be tame, but upon regaining its senses will react quite differently. A case in point was a fox which some small boys found by the side of the road and took home with them. In its dazed condition, apparently from being struck by a car, the animal was quite docile. But as it regained consciousness it reacted naturally and in fright defended itself by biting. I quarantined the animal for about three weeks before releasing it in the mountains.

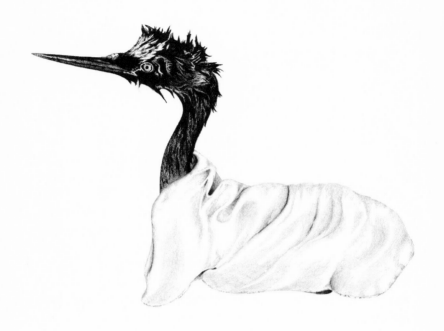

Oiled Grebe

Chapter 8

TREATMENT FOR OIL SPILL
AND
TAR DAMAGE

Oil spills are the greatest threat to the survival of water birds in this increasingly polluted twentieth century. Many pollutants affect wildlife: biocides, heavy metals, manufacturing wastes, urban sewage, and radioactive substances, but crude and refined petroleum spills probably cause more destruction than all other toxins combined.

When oil coats the feathers it weighs down the bird and makes flight difficult or impossible. But oil affects the feather structure itself even more adversely, destroying the waterproofing of individual feathers by disrupting the fine latticework. When a bird can no longer shed water the feathers lose their qualities of insulation and buoyancy. As a result many birds die from chilling, exhaustion and starvation. Ingestion of oil, too, apparently causes the death of many, either by drinking oil-polluted water or by preening oiled feathers. Some of the highly refined types of oil make poisoning a primary hazard to victims of oil spills.

CLEANING

First aid for an oiled bird starts with fresh water, warmth, quiet and darkness. Calm him to reduce stress and to help his system start flushing out the oil which may be permeating it. A rubber band about the beak will keep the bird from preening and further ingesting the toxic substances. Give the bird water as often as possible to flush the gut clean and stop further oil absorption by internal organs.

When an oiled bird arrives at a place where it can be extensively treated, closely inspect the amount of oil damage that has occurred. Heavily oiled birds should be separated from those only lightly affected. Often only small areas of the body need to be cleaned; a glob here or there on the breast or back or under a wing does not require the thorough treatment given a heavily oiled bird.

In cleaning, the less natural oils or waxes removed from the feathers the better. Heavily oiled birds require a more complete cleaning by immersion in or coating with a cleaning agent. At all times be careful not to allow the cleaning agent to get into the eyes, which should be rinsed with clear water, or into the beak. Before washing the beak carefully wrap a rubber band about it to keep the bird from drinking the cleaning solution. Preening may have left an oil coating inside the mouth; offering a smooth stick or a finger usually opens the beak and allows access for cleaning. Cotton swabs soaked with cod liver oil will do the job. Dehydration is a major cause of death in oil-soaked birds, so water should frequently be offered the bird from an eyedropper or basting syringe. Be wary of the sharply pointed beaks of water birds such as grebes, which have a considerable striking radius and can do great damage to human eyes.

At home where one does not have access to the more sophisticated substances used by wildlife veterinarians, mineral oil or a mild dish detergent will often suffice to clean an oiled bird. Mineral oil, which is nontoxic, may necessitate a long stay in captivity, ranging from a few weeks to a few months or even until the next molt, to allow repair of feathers cleaned with this solvent. (When possible a bird should be allowed to molt in his natural environment—molting stresses even the healthiest of birds.) If one uses mineral oil the bird must be toweled dry afterward and kept warm and quiet. If a mild dish detergent is used both the washing solution and the clear water rinse should be warm, just above human body temperature. During washing, the bird's body but not his head should be dipped into the solution or the solution painted on the bird's feathers, swished around gently but thoroughly.

Detergents work well to emulsify oils that are not too tar-like. Some detergents contain fairly toxic substances that may irritate avian skin or, if absorbed through the skin or ingested, damage internal organs. Moreover, the wetting agents found in all detergents can remain on the feathers for weeks causing the plumage to become soaked when the bird enters water. It will therefore be necessary to rinse in warm flowing water until the feathers appear "dry," rinsed free of the wetting agent and able to repel water. This may take up to half an hour. In order not to traumatize the bird, already stressed by his captivity, it may be better to rinse incompletely and allow him a few days' rest in his pen before completing the rinse. During this period don't put a water dish in his pen—give the bird water from a basting syringe, his beak pried open at the base with the fingers. After the bird is able to repel water provide a water dish and a place for bathing under careful supervision to be assured that he does not get a chill.

Mineral oil will do the job but in application of this or any cleaning agent it must be remembered that feathers are easily damaged, and any manipulation other than softly stroking them in their natural direction may result in a rehabilitation time of months instead of days. Always stroke with the "grain." The cleaner will leach out the feathers' natural oils provided by the bird's preen gland. Without sufficient natural oils the feathers soon develop the "frizzies," first at the microscopic level and progressively in the larger structures. Since it is the latticed microstructure and molecular bonding that render a feather water-repellent, even the "micro-frizzies" will cause a feather to soak up water. It is also possible that the preen gland may malfunction due to stress of exhaustion and dousing with cleaning agents.

The microstructure of each feather must be kept skillfully aligned, and the only expert capable of doing so is the bird itself. Good-looking birds have been returned to the wild even though doomed to a chilly death by a progressive case of the "micro-frizzies." People releasing these birds in what appears to be good shape boast of high survival rates without adequately testing how well the birds can support themselves in water. If one has used mineral oil to clean the bird it is important to prevent chilling, which results in a high percentage of deaths among rehabilitated water birds. Start testing with just a few minutes at a time in warm shallow water, followed by toweling dry, and allow him to progress at his own pace. Observe his ability to maintain in the water, how wet his feathers become, how high he floats. The ability to fly is not necessarily an indication of readiness to be released; water birds are often well able to fly before their plumage can repel water. With land birds such as owls and hawks the ability to fly *may* indicate their readiness for release.

To be completely effective a cleaning process would, in addition to removing the oil, restore the waterproofing and insulation of the plumage without any toxic effect while reducing stress to a minimum. Unfortunately no cleaning agent has been found which meets all these necessities. Research has developed such substances as Sol 70, produced by the same companies which spill the oil. One of the cleaning agents used with some success, given the right species and the right type of oil, has been Polycomplex A-11. In the extensive rehabilitation work of the members of International Bird Rescue, Sol 70 has proven to be the most effective so far. There is no all-purpose cleaner, as different kinds of oil require different solvents and different species of birds react differently to various cleaning agents. Fluorocarbon solvents are expensive, and the sophisticated equipment required for their use puts them beyond the scope of home care. Hydrocarbon solvents, though effective in removing even tarlike oil, pose a fire hazard and are toxic. Too, if a bird is at all in poor health or suffering from oil ingestion, a solvent will probably be fatal. For these reasons it is recommended that mineral oil or a mild dish detergent be used. Consult your local wildlife service or Humane Society for further information on the species you are treating and the type of oil encountered.

Reducing stress on the bird to an absolute minimum is extremely important. Often placing a cloth lightly over a bird's head calms him, making the cleaning process easier. Take your time and be diligent to assure the bird a proper and thorough cleaning. If detergent has been used, when rinsing the bird all residue of oil and cleaner must be removed. Turning the bird to permit counterflow of the breast feathers aids flushing. Following rinsing the bird should be patted dry with towels or rags or carefully blown dry with warm air from a hair dryer held not too close. Rest should follow in the warm quiet of a rehabilitation cage or pen.

In the cleaning phase as in the other stages of rescue and rehabilitation gentle handling should be kept foremost in mind. An ornithologist or veterinarian should be consulted as soon as possible.

HOUSING AND FEEDING

In the rehabilitation shelter use a litter of wood shavings or shredded newspapers to prevent aspergillosis. Several inches' thickness of this litter may be necessary for diving birds, who will otherwise drag their bodies and become vulnerable to the development of breast sores, tumors, and bumblefoot. A thinner floor covering may be used for the other types of water and land birds. The litter should be changed daily.

Providing natural food for oiled birds in captivity is often difficult or impossible. Vitamins and some commercial feeds may be of some use, but few commercial feeds meet the minimum daily requirements of wild species. Many of the birds encountered in oil spills require a high protein diet, though this is not as true for, say, dabbling ducks as it would be for grebes, loons, and murres. Dabbling ducks should be fed mash for the first day or so and later cracked grains. Diving ducks should receive mash and a high protein food such as fish and/or brine shrimp for the first few days with cracked grains added later. Shrimp and white bait smelt are available fish seemingly appetizing to these water birds.

A correct diet will be reflected in the condition of the feathers, body weight and general health of the bird. As mentioned previously the molting and replacing of feathers which occurs at least annually for most birds requires a tremendous output of energy and metabolic activity. Only birds in excellent condition seem capable of undergoing this molting process successfully. And it is unfortunately sometimes necessary for a bird to molt after severe feather damage before he may return to the wild. His diet is of prime importance during the molt. The use of live fish is an effective means of stimulating a bird's appetite. Inexperienced handlers should not try force-feeding, which generates considerable stress and often causes other injuries. However, force-feeding may be necessary for some species which will not eat at all unless surrounded by numbers of their own kind. Any wiggling or bait fish from two to seven inches long offered in a pan on the floor or from the hand often induces birds to feed in captivity. Too, birds should always have access to drinking water which is not deep enough for swimming for the first days of captivity, since they might become chilled or otherwise weakened.

I have found the commercially available Terramycin useful in treating cloudy or milky eyes, weight loss, general listlessness and lack of appetite. Dosage of course depends on the size of the bird. Dovekies and teals, for example, require 50 milligrams; scoters and loons require 120 milligrams. It will be necessary to observe the droppings of the bird; diarrhea seems to indicate overdosing. Terramycin is available from most poultry supply houses and veterinarians.

Ointments may help water birds kept in dry surroundings; apply to dry cracking skin on the legs and feet.

RELEASE

The final stage in rehabilitation of these oil-damaged birds is returning them to the wild. If their release is not well-planned all previous efforts may be wasted. Birds cannot simply be turned loose to fend for themselves. A quick change in environment can be traumatic. Birds must acclimate slowly to wild conditions, particularly when they have been in captivity for a long period. Deciding which birds to release and where and when to release them requires considerable attention to each bird. At the very least the feathers must be able to insulate the bird and repel water. A bird's ability to float in water for extended periods of time in the enclosure is a good indication of readiness; particular note should be taken of his buoyancy, how high he rides in the water.

A bird is considered rehabilitated when able to resume normal activities. With water birds normal feeding behavior, preening, and the ability to remain in the water without getting wet to the skin are prerequisites. Dabbling ducks for instance should be able to remain in the water for five minutes without getting wet to the skin before they are ready for release. Diving ducks and cormorants should be able to float for an hour without getting wet to the skin. Such divers as loons, murres, auks, and puffins, and oceanic birds such as the albatross, shearwater, and petrel, should be able to float "dry" for six hours before they are ready to be released. Grebes must be able to remain dry for twenty-four hours in the water before they can be returned to the wild.

An isolated area with sufficient natural foods and cover, relatively free from predation and human disturbance, is an ideal release site. If possible, feed should be provided initially. It may take a few days or longer for birds to become self-sufficient, although I have released birds that had been oil soaked into relatively safe environments such as a lake, pond or quiet backwater and seen them adapt very rapidly. I remember releasing a western grebe who within minutes was diving underwater to feed on the sweet wild fish he had so dearly missed in his months of captivity.

REMOVAL OF TAR

At times birds walk through fresh asphalt or tar on streets or roofs. When it dries it becomes caked on feathers and feet and is very uncomfortable for the bird; if it cakes on the wings, the bird may be unable to fly.

A simple method of removing the tar is with vegetable oil or shortening. Apply the shortening to the tar, allow time for it to penetrate, then remove with tissue. If the tar is quite thick more than one application will be necessary. The shortening not only removes the tar but also acts as a soothing ointment for the flesh.

After the tar has been removed, wash the feathers with a mild detergent and warm water. Be sure not to get the water and detergent into the bird's eyes or mouth.

If the bird has picked at its feathers and gotten tar on its beak, remove with the vegetable shortening but do not wash.

Allow the bird to dry, then feed it and release it.

The above treatment may be used for animals as well.

Chapter 9

TREATMENT FOR ADDITIONAL DISABILITIES

BUMBLEFOOT

Bumblefoot is an inflamed swelling of leg joints all too common with water birds kept in captivity. Because it affects all birds to some degree, one should be cautious in the housing and maintenance of convalescing birds. The condition of bumblefoot is particularly prevalent in diving birds undergoing treatment following oil spills.

Bumblefoot causes a loss of function of the joints which can sometimes be fatal to birds not in the best of health. Diving birds other than auks and penguins rely on feet for propulsion to procure food underwater. They generally need a lengthy run across water or a fall from a cliff to become airborne. Once in the water a lame foot can prevent these divers from regaining the air.

Bumblefoot begins as a swelling of the soft tissues in a leg joint. It is a kind of arthritis which progresses to the harder tissues of cartilage and bone resulting in the immobility of the joint. Symptoms similar to bumblefoot may also occur in wing joints. Treatment with antibiotics rarely seems to be effective, although research is underway to find the best possible medication. Experience has taught that the best treatment is one quarter of a five-grain Bufferin tablet per kilogram per day; though for raptors such as hawks and owls it is not indicated. The Bufferin seems not only to relieve some of the discomfort but also to aid in reducing the swelling, facilitating the bird's natural healing processes.

Watching the conditions that cause abrasion on feet or wings of captive birds is the best preventive measure. Bumblefoot can be caused by a mechanical trauma such as a blow or pressure which causes the primary deterioration that leads to secondary bacterial infection. For birds that spend nearly all their time in the water, merely resting on a hard surface may be sufficiently damaging to the hocks to cause bumblefoot.

MAGGOTS

A maggot is a soft-bodied, grublike, footless larva of an insect, as of the housefly. It is one of the deadliest enemies of the wounded bird or animal during the warm months of the year. The fly is attracted to an open wound, lays its eggs within or around the edge of the wound, and within hours the wound is filled with tiny maggots. An uninjured bird or animal too young to have fur or feathers may also become a hatching place for maggots. Yet repulsive as they may seem, maggots also serve a useful purpose. As the flesh of a wound decays, the maggot feeds upon the dead flesh, thus keeping the wound clean and free of infection. However, unless the wound is discovered and the maggots removed, they will multiply rapidly and eventually penetrate to a vital organ and kill the animal.

Always examine a bird or animal minutely for eggs or maggots, especially if there is any sign of bleeding. Look carefully at the mouth, eyes, ears, and rectal area, and search through the fur or feathers.

The tiny yellow eggs may appear singly or in groups, sometimes constituting clumps as large as the end of your finger. Treatment depends on where eggs or larvae appear, and eyes and ears require very delicate care. If at all possible, take the wounded creature to a veterinarian for removal of the maggots, since he will have certain solutions on hand to cleanse the infected area thoroughly and safely. If the wound is large and the maggots have grown considerably, they may already have done great damage. A veterinarian will recognize the extent of the damage and, if it cannot be successfully treated, will relieve the animal of its suffering. If you must do the job yourself, adhere to the correct procedures for different areas of the body.

The following equipment is required: a glass medicine dropper with a small, rounded end; tweezers; water that has been boiled and cooled to room temperature; penicillin ointment ("refined for eyes only") or a mild eye wash; carbolated salve; cornstarch; peroxide; and white petroleum jelly, mineral oil, or olive oil. You will not need all of the above for every area, but select what is needed per the directions.

The patient will need to be immobilized during treatment. Wrap him in gauze or a towel, depending on his size and strength, exposing only the area to be treated. Be sure the nostrils are not covered so that the patient may breathe freely. Have all the equipment assembled on a table in front of you before you immobilize the creature.

Maggot Removal—Eyes and Ears

Never use tweezers on the eyes—use only the medicine dropper. Metal tweezers might cut or jab the eyes, whereas the smooth end of a medicine dropper will do no harm if used gently.

Partly fill two glasses with sterilized water. One glass will contain the water you are going to drop into the eye; use the other glass of water to dispose of the maggots. Drop a few drops of water into the eye and then suck the water back up into the dropper. If the maggots are small enough to go through the end of the dropper they can be disposed of in the second glass of water. If they are too large to go into the dropper, the suction will hold them against the end of the dropper for disposal. You will probably get only one maggot at a time so the process will have to be repeated until all are removed. These creatures move very fast, but the repeated dropping of water into the eye usually washes them into the corners where they are accessible to the dropper.

After all maggots have been removed, treat the eye with the penicillin ointment or a mild eye wash. Do not use any other kind of medicine on the eyes unless it is specified by a veterinarian. It is better to use nothing at all than something that might injure the eye. I have used this method many times with no apparent damage. Examine the patient several times a day until you are sure that you have removed all of the maggots and that no new ones have hatched.

Use the same method for removal of maggots from the ears. I have used tweezers in the ears, but *only* when the maggots were close to the surface and large enough to be easily captured without injury to the ear.

Maggot Removal—Body Wounds

On body wounds I have found that flushing the wound with peroxide is effective. Sometimes in removing maggots from superficial wounds it will suffice to coat the area heavily with cornstarch. Maggots need to be wet to move freely, and when the coat of cornstarch dries they drop off.

After removing maggots from a body wound apply carbolated salve thoroughly to the wound. This disinfects and helps the healing process. (Do not use carbolated salve in or around the mouth or eyes.)

For removing the eggs before they have a chance to hatch, use tissue or gauze saturated in white petroleum jelly, mineral oil, or olive oil.

Again, I would like to stress the importance of using great care in working in and around the eyes. Keep a careful watch for a few days to be absolutely certain that you have removed all of the maggots and that no new eggs have hatched.

CUTEREGRA

Cuteregra eggs are laid on rabbits, rats, etc. by a fly which develops into a worm which nests in the skin. As the growing larva nourishes itself on the body of the host, the hole in the skin of the animal enlarges. These worms are commonly called "worbles." I removed as many as a dozen, the size of my little finger, from the body of a large Belgian hare. They are easy to remove and the treatment of the animal afterwards is simple. Go over the body of the animal minutely and locate each sore and remove the larvae with tweezers. Have a glass of disinfectant at hand—alcohol, peroxide, or Phisohex—and apply it with a medicine dropper to wash out the vacated wound. The animal should be examined carefully each day to locate any new larvae that may develop and also to clean and disinfect the old wounds. Be especially diligent in examining the area of the testicles on a male animal. I would suggest keeping the animal confined to bug-free quarters for a period of at least two weeks to be sure no new larvae develop.

MITES

These little pests are not confined to chickens and sparrows—any bird may have them. You can remove them with very little effort by using a type of powder manufactured expressly for mites on birds. Tear a hole in a piece of tissue or paper towel, insert the bird's head. In this way you will protect the eyes, mouth and nostrils of the bird from the powder. Dust the powder freely through the feathers, being sure to get the powder under the wings and around the neck area. Remove the paper from the bird's head and release it into a cage or box whose floor has been lined with paper towels. By using white paper on the floor of the cage you can see just how many mites fall off, and the paper can be removed and burned as it becomes soiled.

Always keep birds under treatment segregated from birds with no mites. It is a good idea to isolate any new bird for a few days until you are sure he is free of vermin. Sometimes the warmth of your hands as you hold a bird will cause the mites to crawl off onto you, but soap and water will remove them.

Flea powder may also work for removal of mites on larger birds, but I do not recommend this as it might be too strong and kill the bird. It is best to get a powder that is made especially for birds. Cages that have become infested with mites should be sprayed with chlordane, then washed with a detergent, scalded, and thoroughly dried before using again.

FLAT FLIES (FEATHER LICE)

A type of fly may be found on hawks, owls and pigeons that is as large as a house fly but of a different shape. Their bodies are flat in appearance and the wings fan out, and they move swiftly from side to side through the feathers of a bird. A falconer tells me they are usually found on all birds, apparently do no harm to the bird, and will not stay on the bird long. I mention them only so that you will not be alarmed upon discovering them on a bird.

TRIMMING BEAKS AND TOENAILS

All animals and birds in captivity need to have their toenails and/or beaks trimmed. In the natural state their constant foraging for survival creates the wear that counteracts overgrowth of beaks and nails.

Trimming of beaks and toenails should be done cautiously to avoid bleeding; it is best to take off just a little at a time rather than cut too much and injure the bird or animal.

Sometimes a bird's beak will grow so long that it hampers the feeding process, and the ends may cross, making it impossible to pick up food. Toenails which have grown too long will catch on the wires of a cage, and the bird's struggling can cause injury as serious as a broken leg.

Scissors, small but heavy enough to cut through the tough substance of the beak or toenail, are best for this purpose. After the main portion has been cut away, use an emery board to file any rough edges. Usually the dead portion of the beak or toenail is easily distinguished from the live area by its color. It will also appear dry and scaly. Only this part should be removed.

Chapter 10

PETS VS. WILDLIFE

CATS

Very few birds or animals caught by cats survive. They may escape, but most die of injuries and shock. The long sharp teeth and claws of a cat, while making a very small wound, usually penetrate deep into the body of the prey injuring vital organs or causing a fatal infection.

A cat or dog allowed to roam is a nuisance to those who love birds and like to feed them in their yard. The cat allowed to roam who has not been spayed or altered contributes to the overflow of kittens destroyed by the thousands in animal shelters each year.

Cats do not need to roam to be happy; this has been proven many times over by responsible individuals who cherish their cats. Cats loose at night are a menace to baby birds and small wild animals. A bell about a cat's neck is of no aid to a bird too young to fly: the belled cat needs no stealth to destroy ground nests and helpless baby birds.

Those cat owners who refuse to bring an unwanted cat to the animal shelter, choosing instead to abandon their pet in the countryside, are cruel and irresponsible. This "giving the cat a chance" usually results, for the cat, in bewilderment, hunger, disease, danger from wild animals or dogs, exposure to the elements, and in the case of an unspayed female probably a litter of kittens to add to the growing menace of half-wild predators.

PET SHOPS

During the years that I was Humane Agent for the Animal Welfare League in Arlington and Fairfax counties in Virginia, I saw many pet shops which lacked proper facilities—hawks and other large birds confined in cages so small they could not stretch their wings; monkeys and other furred animals caged in the same restrictive manner and often sitting in their own wastes. Monkeys become paralyzed if not exercised. They are affectionate, but because they cannot be housebroken they seldom make good pets.

I recall an instance where a huge shopping center had as part of their decor a large cage where birds moved about in seeming freedom. But the place was artificially lighted and the cement floor was always wet. I saw beautiful pheasants walking aimlessly around picking at the wet cement in search of something to eat. I was told that the turnover of birds was considerable, and that if one died it was quickly replaced by another. What a poor life for these wildlings, but better than in a pet shop in the same shopping center where the birds were placed on tables between the aisles and exposed to the poking fingers of the public.

I have found sick birds put in boxes in back rooms and left to die. I have seen canaries in such filth that their feet were balled with droppings and they could not perch. Once I was called to inspect birds in a dime store where they had been left over a weekend without care. There were as many as thirty-five parakeets to a cage, with dry water cups and no food. When I called attention to their condition the clerk derided me, so I opened new boxes of food and emptied them onto the floor of the cages. The birds literally dropped from their perches to get the seed. These cages were much too small for so many birds and the water cups were of the open type and placed beneath the perches so that the water was soon clouded with droppings.

The selling of such wild animals as skunks, raccoons, and

foxes by either pet stores or private individuals should be prohibited. Skunks de-scented by animal brokers and thus deprived of their natural means of defense can never return to the wild. Raccoons may become virtual vegetables if kept in captivity too long; some become mean and have to be destroyed.

At the present time I am caring for two birds which should never have been removed from their native region. A Savannah hawk, a ward of the state of Virginia, was turned over to me by a game warden. With no toes on either foot, this beautiful bird must be cared for throughout his lifetime. A Hyacinth jay, beautiful and wild, I bought from a pet shop after months of watching him mope about his small cage.

A functional and humane pet shop should provide facilities for all the pets, suitable to each species' needs. For airborne birds this would include sizable flight cages with perches of a size to fit the particular bird's feet comfortably, or varied sizes if more than one type of bird is housed in one cage. The shop would see to proper placing of water cups and feed dishes so that the droppings do not get into them.

Cages for animals should be large enough so that they can exercise and do not have to stand in their own filth. Water dishes and feed dishes should be firmly secured to the sides of the cages. Bedding should be on a raised portion of the cage where it won't get wet or dirty.

For monkeys and all climbing animals ample limbs and perches should be supplied so the animal can stretch and exercise himself and get above his droppings.

All cages should be behind glass or wire so there is no chance for customers to poke at or otherwise annoy the creatures. This is also insurance against colds and diseases that might be transmitted to the animals. At least a counter should be between animal and customer. The store should be lighted in such a way that an animal or bird can get away from glaring light bulbs.

All cages should be positioned so that a bird or animal can get out of drafts (never on the floor). This could be accomplished by placing glass between the cages if they are against a wall or solid backdrop, or by placing glass along the backs and one side of each cage so that a draftless corner is formed. A moderate temperature should be maintained in the store at all times. I have seen birds huddled together in the bottom of cages where air conditioning was too cold for them and no attempt had been made to cover two sides of the cage to prevent the circulating air from blowing on the birds.

All cages and pens should be cleaned daily. Each enclosure should be cleaned and disinfected before any new creature is released into it. Thought should be given to supplying each creature with treats in food other than just the daily minimum diet of the same old foods.

There are many pet shops which maintain a high degree of responsibility in dealing with their charges and which do not equate life with financial profit. It is to those few grossly negligent stores that this section is dedicated. I have known shops to offer full authenticated information on the feeding and care of each pet they sold, and from them I have learned that the business of selling pets can be conducted humanely.

Chapter 11

PREPARING FOR RELEASE

The timing of release is critical to the survival of a young bird or animal. Reluctance to release is evidence that the creature is being subjected to personal feelings rather than true consideration. The person who pampers, pets and confines a wild creature to the point where it is unable to adjust to its wild state is not a friend to that creature. The parent who lets a child imprison a wild creature as a plaything until it weakens and dies is guilty of an unjust and inhumane attitude toward both the imprisoned wildling and the child. A wild creature should be kept confined only as long as it really needs help; then it should be released, and your attention should be turned to another which may need your services.

The migratory birds are especially harmed by being kept in captivity too long. These birds need to be released as soon as possible so that they can condition themselves for the ardors of migration. Often a bird need only be helped overnight, as with grebes who land in a city and cannot take off from solid ground. There are also those longer visiting grebes who, having spied light shimmering on macadam mistakenly attempt to land and break a leg.

The importance of releasing birds unable to fly even in an aviary has been proven many times. Since these birds stay around for days getting handouts and moving freely on the ground, in shrubs and in trees, they develop better feathers and learn to exercise wings that previously hung low and out of place, and eventually learn to fly. If they are kept too long in captivity, where they can only hop short distances, they may not develop the ability to fly. But beware of cats in your area.

The best place of release is where the bird or animal has been raised, if possible. If natural hazards seem too great, however, it is best to locate a home in a remote and safe area where the animal or bird may be kept in captivity for a few days to acclimate to the new surroundings, and then released. Do not release birds into a room which does not have curtains over the windows, since they may try to fly out and thereby injure themselves against the glass.

Some people have raised raccoons, opossums, squirrels and other wild animals in the middle of large housing developments. Naturally it is impossible to release these animals in such areas. It is necessary to find natural wild areas. Many such creatures have been brought to me. Some were placed on large estates where animals of the same species were found in the wild, and where a person was present who would foster the transition to the wild. The most thoughtless thing I can imagine is raising a baby raccoon and making it dependent on human care, and then, without prior adjustment, leaving the confused creature in an unfamiliar area. Even though wild cousins may live nearby, the first instinct is to head for the nearest human dwelling. Trusting humans because they are the only parents he knows, the poor little fellow is shot, trapped, or hunted by dogs.

I prefer to release birds from an outside aviary. This can be done anywhere, even in a housing development, except with some species. Obviously, water birds need their own environment. Owls and hawks need another type of releasing situation. The young hawk I wintered over because I doubted he would survive the winter on his own has been free for weeks and still comes around every other day for a handout. He perches on the fence between the house and garage, patiently waiting for me to feed him. I always know he has arrived when the grackles and robins set up an awful din. All the time he is eating he keeps up a conversation and when finished arranges himself on the fence to preen and sun. I've put a chunk of firewood down to place his food on. If I offer a choice tidbit like a dead mouse, he pounces on it with gusto, and characteristic of hawks spreads his wings to hide his kill, all the time protesting with that squeaky little voice. I hope he reverts to the wild by fall, otherwise I will have to haul him into the aviary again for the winter. For the most part, birds can be released at home where they can come and go at will during the daytime and rest safely at night until accustomed to living in the wild. Usually these young creatures move about freely during the day, coming in now and then for food to supplement what they are able to find for themselves, and in the late afternoon returning to the aviary for the night. This place denotes food and safety to them. As they become stronger, they may still come in for handouts but will probably elect to sleep outside. This is the day you have waited for: they have become self-sufficient and free to be the wild creatures they were meant to be.

The individual who raises a bird or animal and then suddenly releases and ignores it is doing the creature a great disservice. A young bird will depend on the parent bird for help until it is as large as the parent. In lieu of natural parents, the person who raises it becomes the source of food and a haven of safety. If the bird or animal is taken abruptly to a strange place and released, it may become very confused; and since it has been sheltered, may not adequately recognize danger, thus decreasing its chance of survival. The alert and wary wild creature is the one with the best chance of survival, and a too trusting creature often does not survive the intense predator/prey relationships of the wild.

You may have great attachment to the creatures you are raising. I have certainly enjoyed every bird and animal I have cared for. I have been fascinated by the personality differences in many of the same species, amused by their antics during growth, and worried, as many a mother, when they asserted their independence and disappeared from my world altogether. I've always been careful not to make pets of any of them, making them too tame or trusting. In fact, I seldom even attach a nickname to them. Inevitably, there are those whose manner or disability invites a name, such as the robin brought to me with a gash on its skull caused by a tumble from the nest or a peck from a grackle or blue jay. The feathers never covered this wound, so he ended up being called "Baldy."

Kindness, a gentle voice, slow movements that won't frighten, and careful handling are always necessary. But avoid the temptation to caress, fondle or domesticate wild animals or birds.

If you are going to take the time to raise a wild creature, then also take the time to help him adjust to new surroundings, new sounds and smells. Patience will be needed; some of your charges will respond almost immediately, but others may take days or even weeks.

IDENTIFICATION AND BANDING

Positive identification is required before a bird can be banded by a licensed bander of the government's Fish and Wildlife Service. If you do not know of a bander in your area, write to the Fish and Wildlife Service in Washington, D.C., for information.

Banded birds furnish help to the government in researching migratory habits, life span, and other characteristics. The band is also a positive means of determining whether a bird you have raised returns periodically or stays in your area after release.

If you find a dead bird with a band imprinted with a number, the letters F and W, and "Wash. D.C." on it, either return the band to the Fish and Wildlife Service, Interior Department, Washington, D.C., or send them the band number. Identify the bird if possible, state where and when found, and include your name and address. You will receive a card from the agency giving the bird's identity and banding history.

BIBLIOGRAPHY

Arbib, Robert. *Hungry Bird Book*. New York: Ballantine, 1972.

Clark, R. B. "Oil Pollution and the Conservation of Seabirds," Int'l Conf. on Oil Pollution of the Sea (Rome), Paper No. 5, page 76, October 1968.

Clark, R. B. and Kennedy, J. R. *How Oiled Seabirds Are Cleaned*. Newcastle Upon Tyne: University of Newcastle Upon Tyne, 1971.

Clark, R. B. and Kennedy, J. R. *Rehabilitation of Oiled Seabirds*. Newcastle Upon Tyne: University of Newcastle Upon Tyne, 1968.

Davis, Anderson, Karstead, Trainer, eds. *Infectious and Parasitic Diseases of Wild Birds*. Ames, Iowa: The Iowa State University Press, 1971.

Department of the Interior. *Review of the Problem of Birds Contaminated by Oil and Their Rehabilitation*. Washington, D.C.: U.S. Government Printing Office, 1970.

Department of the Interior and Department of Transportation. *Oil Pollution*. Washington, D.C.: U.S. Government Printing Office, 1968.

Dossenbach, Hans D. and Buhrer, Emil M. *The Family Life of Birds*. San Francisco, California: McGraw-Hill Book Co., 1971.

Environmental Protection Agency. *Effects of Oil Pollution on Waterfowl —A Study of Salvage Methods*. Washington, D.C.: U.S. Government Printing Office, 1970.

Levine, Stephen. *Planet Steward: A Journal of Days and Species*. San Francisco, California: Unity Press, 1973.

Marshall, A. J. *Biology and Comparative Physiology of Birds (2 Vols.)* New York: Academic Press, 1960.

Martin, Alexander C., Zim, Herbert S., and Nelson, Arnold L. *American Wildlife and Plants, A Guide to Wildlife Food Habits.* New York: Dover Publications, 1951.

McLeod, W. M., Trotter, D. M., and Lumb, J. W., *Avian Anatomy.* Minneapolis, Minnesota: Burgess Publishing Co., 1964.

Pearson, T. Gilbert. *Birds of America.* Garden City, New York: Doubleday & Co., 1936.

Peterson, Roger Tory. *A Field Guide to Birds.* Boston, Massachusetts: Houghton Mifflin Co., 1969.

Robbins, C. S., Bruun, B., and Zim, H. S. *Birds of North America: A Guide to Field Identification.* New York: Golden Press, 1966.

Smith, David. International Bird Rescue Newsletter (Vol. 1-4). Berkeley, California, 1972

Smith, David. Letter to Royal Forest and Bird Protection Society of New Zealand, *Re* Treatments for Oil Spill Damage. International Bird Rescue Research Center. Berkeley, California, April 1973.

Stanton, Philip B. *A Bibliography, Operation Rescue.* Washington, D.C.: American Petroleum Institute, 1972.

Stanton, Philip B. *Operation Rescue.* Washington, D.C.: American Petroleum Institute, 1972.

Terres, John K. *Songbirds in Your Garden.* New York: Thomas Y. Crowell Co.

Thomas, Arline. *Bird Ambulance.* New York: Bantam, 1971.

Van Tyne, J. and Berger, A. *Fundamentals of Ornithology.* New York: Dover Publications, 1971.

Welty, Joel Carl. *The Life of Birds.* Philadelphia: S. B. Saunders Co., 1962.

BIOGRAPHICAL NOTES

Mae Hickman was born in Kansas in 1907 to pioneer parents who homesteaded the Fox Strip of Oklahoma. The youngest of ten children, she was placed in a foster home at four months old when her mother died. The first seven years of her life were spent on a large western ranch where no other children lived, and there her affinity for animals developed. She returned to live with her father and family until age sixteen, when she left to attend school in Florida. She married in 1926, moved to Virginia, and since then has continued to work with wildlife at home while raising four children.

Maxine Guy graduated from the University of Nebraska as an art major and attended the Chicago Art Institute, leaving to work at Marshall Fields in Chicago. She entered the U.S. Army in 1942 with the first officer candidate group of the Women's Army Corps, and served as a captain and division chief on General MacArthur's staff during the postwar occupation of Japan. She was married to an army officer and has been an army wife until recently. A professional potter who has studied at several eastern universities and art institutes, she spends much of her time at work in her ceramic studio, The Potted Owl, in Tubac, Arizona. Behind the studio, with the aid of the local townspeople, she has completed a remarkable system of outdoor aviaries where she continues to help the furred and feathered.

David Haskins, originally of Massachusetts, is presently studying art at the University of California at Berkeley and lives in Larkspur with his lady Susan. A former student of Alton Raible, he has become proficient in expressing his continuous involvement with wildlife. This is his first series of book illustrations.

INDEX

Oh cage me not, lest I become a prisoner to man's ego
Deny me not my right to fly in God's blue sky
and spy upon those mortals there below
That when I see a friend, I may descend to serenade
And when my song is o'er, away on freedom's wings
to soar

MAE HICKMAN